"Since *everyone* is impacted by cancer in some way, this book should be read by and shared with *everyone*. In these pages, Abigail shares her innermost thoughts of watching her baby deal with cancer, and I wasn't prepared for the personal impact it would have on me. It reminded me how to minister to and pray for those who are part of this horrible disease. Most importantly, it renewed my understanding of how to endure hardship with God's help. I am reminded again that God is good all the time."

—Terry Lancaster, Wife of Bob (Multiple Myeloma), Founder of the Cotinga Foundation, Special Ed Teacher

"This honest, transparent, deeply-revealing story of a mother walking through the depths with her child has blessed us beautifully. The book is addressed to mothers who are also walking with a child through cancer, but it speaks to everyone who loves and cares. Abigail's depth of trust in God strengthens my faith, and I believe it will yours."

—Clyde and Elaine Meador, Former Vice President and Wife for the International Mission Board

"Scripture encourages us to comfort others with the comfort we have received from the God of compassion and care. Robert and Abigail freely share their beautifully chronicled journey with a desire to help others who may be walking the difficult road they've traveled with their precious daughter, Esther. Their example is powerful, their story is inspirational, and their faith in God is their foundation."

—Jon and Sarah Young, Lead Pastor and Wife, Dayton Avenue Baptist Church, Xenia, OH

"Abigail's book puts words to many of the thoughts and emotions I had during my son's illness. Her sentiments about prayer and family spoke to my heart and showed a profound wisdom gifted to her by God. Well done."

—Joni Flora, Parent to Thomas (fighting AML)

"The Cancer Moms Club is one that nobody wants to join, yet Abigail Walker shares her heart and experiences in this club with genuine grace, honesty, humility, humor, and hope. As we follow Abigail's precious daughter's leukemia journey in her book, we learn through her gentle but truthful explanations and stories that even though cancer in our children can be an awful and devastating roller coaster, God provides the strength, hope, and guidance for each moment of each day. We encounter a kind and caring friend in these pages, and Abigail also points to the kind and caring Friend who is ultimately in control when our lives seem upended by our children's cancer diagnosis."

—Rose Waligora, Cancer Mom to Eric (T-ALL, 2014–2017 active treatments)

SUFFERING, ENDURANCE, CHARACTER & HOPE

A STORY OF PEDIATRIC CANCER AND A MOTHER'S LOVE

Abigail Walker

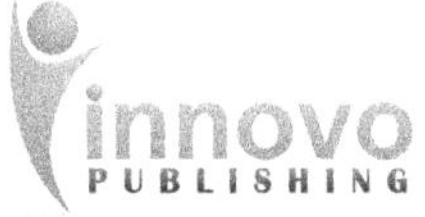

Published by Innovo Publishing, LLC
www.innovopublishing.com
1-888-546-2111

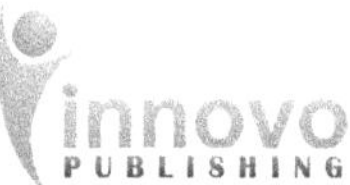

Providing Full-Service Publishing Services for Christian Authors,
Artists & Ministries:
Books, eBooks, Audiobooks, Music, Screenplays, Film & Courses

SUFFERING, ENDURANCE, CHARACTER & HOPE
A Story of Pediatric Cancer and a Mother's Love

Certain names used by permission. All other personal names have been altered to protect the privacy of the individuals.

Library of Congress Control Number: 2020941954
ISBN: 978-1-61314-538-8

Cover Design & Interior Layout: Innovo Publishing, LLC

Printed in the United States of America
U.S. Printing History
First Edition: 2020

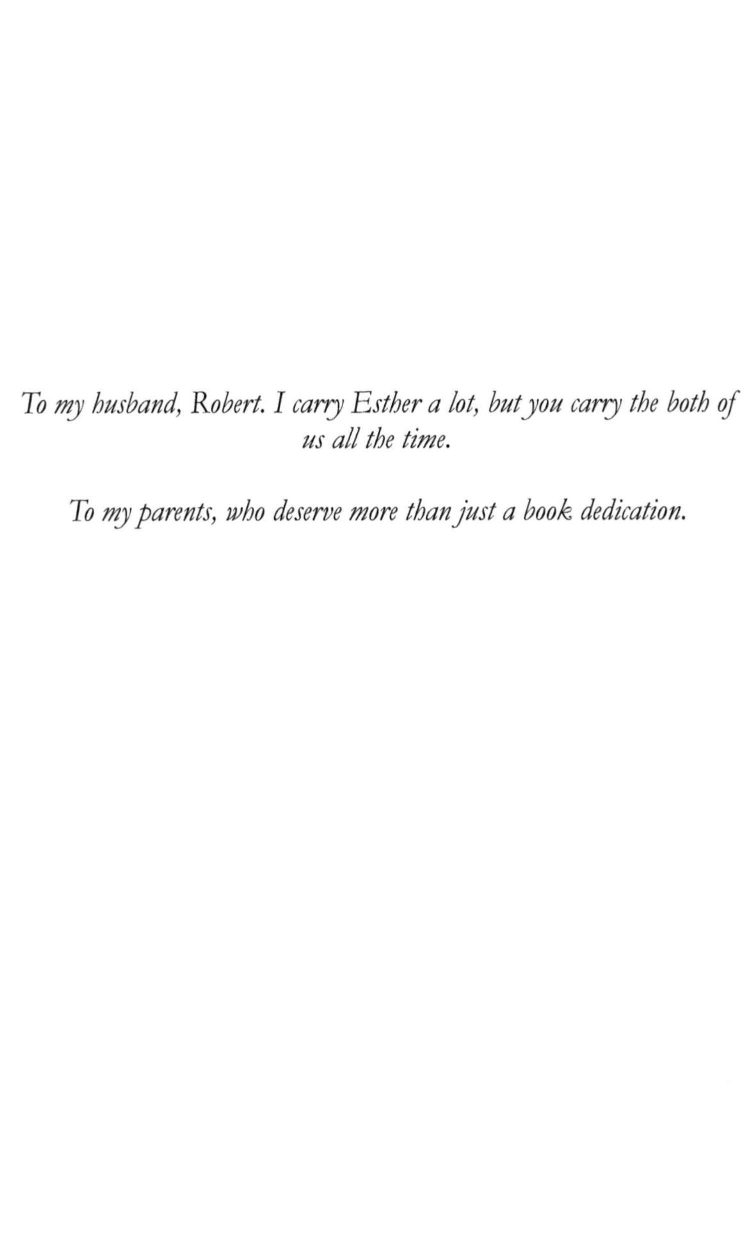

To my husband, Robert. I carry Esther a lot, but you carry the both of us all the time.

To my parents, who deserve more than just a book dedication.

Contents

Foreword

Children are a blessing. This is what I mutter under my breath as I stare in horror at the war-torn, ravaged remains of what used to be a tidy home—about five years ago before the first bundle of chaos was birthed. I stand there with arms crossed, trying to appear calm and firm as my three-year-old finishes his tantrum on the living room floor, but all I want to do is weep at what appears to be my own failure as a mother. I want to close my eyes and rest for a few minutes, to recharge for what will assuredly come that day—but today is the day my three children decided they've all outgrown naptime and cannot seem to find a moment of entertainment from even *one toy in the mound*, complaining that they are "bored."

The prayers of a mother are echoed throughout the world: "Lord, please protect my children from harm." Amidst the chaos and frustration of the day to day, this prayer stands. Because even though parenting is hard, we realize that yes, *children are a blessing.* And all a mother wants is for her children to grow up and thrive in this world. But for some mothers, God decides to give them a different story.

"Your child has cancer" is probably near the top of the nightmare list for parents. The dreams and plans that you have for your family and your child's future all flash in horrific time-lapse through your mind. Not just the unknown future, but the unknown present becomes petrifying—a freeze frame of fear. As a parent, to let your mind wander to *what could happen* could all but paralyze you.

Esther's diagnosis was shared during our Monday night small group, and the news pierced my heart as if it was given to *me*. My soul wretched over what my dear friend was going through as she held her tiny, perfect daughter and relived over and over the moment she received the call. *How will she get through this? How will she be the strength her tiny daughter needs to help her fight this battle—when there's no promised happy ending?*

As a mother of three very young children, I'm not unlike every other mother who constantly worries about her children's safety. My mind races on a continuous "what if" cycle of anxiousness and how I can most protect them from harm. But cancer is a whole other beast. It sweeps through in the middle of the night and catches hold of your loved one, often without warning. It *knows* that you can't stop it. That you couldn't have done anything to prevent it. And yes, God allows it.

As I studied a photo of this little girl whose face still held features of infancy, I thought, *Her body is just so small. How can she possibly fight this on her own?* And what I've seen through my dear friend's journey is the remarkable strength and endurance that can only be credited to a Father who sustains through trials. Oh, how she would just long for a day of "normalcy" that so many parents complain about. But *these* are the days she's been given, and God has continued to be good.

There are days when the chaos around me causes me to cry out, *Why, God? When will these children learn?* But the cries of a mother as she lays with her child in a hospital bed, tucking the wisps of hair behind her daughter's ear as she prays for just a little more time, cause me to pause. The reality that "children are a blessing" becomes raw and real. Time is precious. Clutter can be cleaned. Discipline can be handed out. Gratefulness can be taught. But the long days we have with our children are what we will praise God for in the end. No matter how many days or years we are given with them on this earth, I want to be thankful. Because they could be taken from me at any moment, and all I'd have left are my memories of that messy room, the tiny stomping feet, and the bored expressions—and I'd be praying for *just one more of those days.*

—Rachael Carrington
A mother and a friend

Preface

My friend,

If you're reading this because your little one has cancer, we have too much in common. It doesn't matter that I have a toddler with leukemia, and you have a teenager with a brain tumor; we are now linked by common experience, bonded by trauma. We are different people with different lives and ways of processing things, and as individuals, we see the world in our own unique way. My journey is not your journey; we can draw parallels between them, but there is no exact fit.

We love our children fiercely and would sacrifice just about anything for them. Seeing them go through this incredibly difficult time is likely the worst period of your life. Believe me, I know. But that doesn't mean good can't come out of it.

I am hopeful that my story and my tidbits of advice (I am not brave enough nor mature enough to call it wisdom) will be helpful to you. I want you to not feel alone. The most rewarding part of this trip down the rabbit hole, outside of the healing process of my child and the growth I have experienced in Father God, has been standing alongside other parents. Strong women and men. Fellow warriors in this unwanted battle.

My desire is that through these pages, you will be encouraged by my meager enlightenment on the subject of caring for a loved one with cancer. I have unwittingly begun to be an expert in this field.

I am still making it, and you will too. Take it one day at a time. Give yourself grace.

Much love,

Abigail

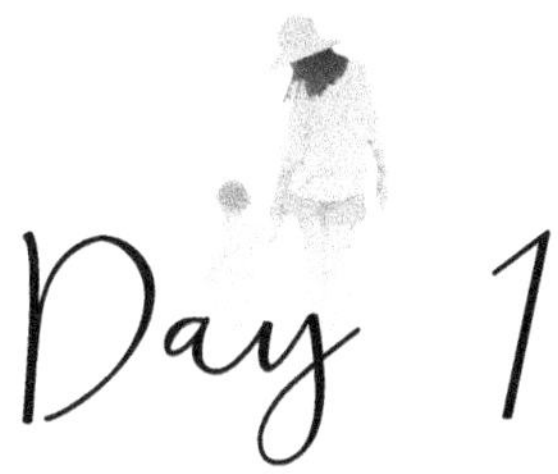

Day 1

Nobody expects it.

On Wednesday, my barely twelve-month-old, who had been walking for over a month, suddenly stopped walking. She was a very active child who loved every step of development she gained, but she had reverted back to crawling (or just sitting). Observing this as her mother, this was concerning. So on Thursday, I took her to her pediatrician. She suspected Esther's cold was inflaming her joints and making it painful to walk. Regardless, she sent me to get her hip X-rays and a blood test. On Friday, she sent for more blood tests.

Maybe that should have been a clue.

Then over the weekend, my baby started walking again! But the rejoicing we had over her seeming "return to normalcy" would quickly be shaken by what happened the next day.

On Monday, October 15, 2018, Esther's doctor called. I was just about to put my child down for a nap. She was melting down around my ankles—something that I would have no strength but to find myself doing moments later.

People describe shock in a variety of metaphors. "Hit them like a ton of bricks." "Blew them away." "Shell shocked." But when our pediatrician said, "Your daughter likely has leukemia," the floor fell out from beneath me. The ground swallowed me whole, and I can still point to the spot on the living room floor where the carpet gave way and sent me careening into the earth.

Leukemia. That's not possible. How could that be? It has to be a mistake, I thought.

I held my swirling thoughts and questions and tears in just long enough to finish the necessary conversation. When I hung up the phone, I staggered up the stairs, carrying my understandably sobbing child. My perfect child. Only twelve months old. Once I reached the top, I immediately dialed my husband, Robert. Breathless, in ragged, choked sobs, I burst out with the earth-shattering words that I didn't even believe myself. I had to repeat myself twice to make him understand. It might've been my incomprehensibility, but it also could have easily been the two-ton brick I just threw in his face. Regardless, the man is a pillar of strength. He was, as always, calm, collected. A safe refuge for me when the world was falling apart. He came straight home to me to fix what he could fix, and to be a haven of stability for what he could not.

Leukemia is bad. What does that entail? What treatment does she get? Chemotherapy? Radiation? Surgery? Can I donate my bone marrow? She and I are the same blood type. That has to count for something. All these thoughts chased through my head as I settled my baby against my breast to nap, waiting for Robert to return home. Esther's breaths turned deep and calm. I could not say the same for mine. Tears rolled down my face, unchecked, and I struggled to contain the sobs pressed tightly to the backs of my eyelids as I gave my child her last nap of an era: the pre-cancer era.

While gazing down at my precious baby, so safe and warm in my arms, I tried not to dwell on the one question that any other mother would notice I left out. *Will my child live?* But I failed in that attempt. It consumed my mind in the quiet of the room, as my fear leaked out of the corners of my eyes and left streams down my face. *What will I do? I'm not strong enough. God, I'm not strong enough!*

The phrase "crying out to God" had never resonated so fully with me before. It's all I could verbalize from the voice in my head. *I'm not strong enough! I'm not strong enough! Oh, Father God! Please!* In the midst of my anguish, the first of many good things to come out of this experience happened. God spoke to me. It was so clear that it was as if He spoke it out loud (but I suppose I'm thankful He didn't, because it would have woken my child up).

"But I Am. *You* are *not* strong enough. But I Am."

My crying slowed to a trickle. My thoughts and fears did not stop, but there was something of peace that moved through me in that moment. Then my husband came in the room where I held our tiny daughter, and he held me—he held both of us in his warm, comforting arms. We shared a few moments in shared grief. A moment of holy sorrow over the fallen world we live in, that it touches things we love the most and taints them—including my small, perfect, barely one-year-old daughter.

And it began. The journey. Oh, how I hate that word, and how I've tried never to use it. But it's hard to avoid. What a word. It sounds like we were visiting the Grand Canyon and things went wrong. It's a word people use with serious illness to make things sound upbeat and peppy.

Believe me, nothing about this is peppy.

***

> ## Oct 15
>
> Nobody wants to make this post. We're currently at Dayton Children's, where Esther is scheduled for a biopsy in the morning. Bloodwork is almost certainly pointing to leukemia. Please pray for us. God is still good in the midst of the bad. We pray this time of hardship for us will point others to Him.

Before we went to the hospital to get more answers to begin Esther's treatment plan, another good thing happened. Our pastor and his wife came to visit us. They are two of the kindest, most caring individuals I have ever known. My husband had been serving as children's pastor at our church for the past year and a half, so we had come to know Pastor Jon and Sarah well. And they were there for us the moment we were thrown into the whirlwind. The leaders of the church who set the pace that the rest of our church family would follow.

They gathered us together in their arms, encompassing our bodies and our souls in a group hug that seemed to lighten the load just a little bit. I cried as we huddled, a circle of prayer and compassion. Esther snuggled close to me as I held her, with not even a faintness of understanding. I shielded her from the tears that dripped slowly off my cheeks.

The specific words that Pastor and his sweet wife used are lost to time in my memory. But the general idea remained: hope in the midst of uncertainty. Faith in our God who brings good in the midst of bad. A deep caring of our church family for our wellbeing. It was only a few minutes, but it was a moment of calm clarity we didn't know we needed. And it served as a foundation for where we would take our next steps into this unknown.

***

We packed our hospital bags, feeling that at any moment we would wake up from this dream. As we drove the thirty minutes to the hospital, the sounds of our GPS along with mundane conversations like, "Watch out for that car! There's clearly a crazy person driving it" filled the air. It felt surreal. It felt like we should be in an ambulance, or in a processional, or have our hazard lights on—something to alert those around us that everything was not all right.

We arrived at the hospital and had to check in at the front desk. *A photo ID, really?* I would say having our photo taken in that moment was as unfortunate as having a driver's license photo taken, except it's a deep step down from there. Something more akin to a Sam's Club® ID. The camera points up your nose, and you're really not certain if this is an appropriate time to stare stoically or to smile (if you are even able). And the best part about this photo, taken on the worst day of your life, is that you get to wear that confused and distressed face on your chest every blessed day for the rest of your life—or time in the hospital.

#blessed.

We made our way up the elevator, stepping off to the fourth floor for the first time of what would be countless. "Hematology/Oncology," I read.

But that's where kids with cancer go.

Oh yeah, that's my kid.

I'd like to say I was noting every facial expression of my child at this point; watching her on the cusp of this enormous life change. Checking on how she was feeling. Attending to her needs. But the truth is, when I looked down at her, nestled safely between my arm and my hip, all I could feel was a selfish, blind terror. I made sure she was still safe in my arms and that she hadn't snuck away to poison the cancer out of her system when I wasn't paying attention. The hammer stroke to her life had not fallen yet; she didn't know everything was about to change

But I did. This was my time of realization and floundering to come upright. I needed her in my arms to keep me from going under. I had to keep her close to keep myself strong. Or at least, as strong as I could be as a mother of a baby with cancer.

The tears welled up again, and I hoped nobody noticed. But I assumed people cried all the time here, so what did it matter?

We were ushered into a small room in what felt like a maze of a department. They weighed and measured my child, taking her blood pressure and her temperature. This is something that would become routine in my future, but in the present, I was terrified as I watched them do these things. And my poor, confused baby cried. *If she can't handle these, how will she handle much worse?*

"Just a little hug!" said the lady in scrubs, putting the minuscule blood pressure cuff on Esther's leg. "Just tickling your forehead!" She ran the thermometer across her tiny little forehead.

My child wailed. She didn't understand this soothing language. I was irrationally angry at this lady for not recognizing this. *Just get it over with!* I thought.

Then the doctor came in. He introduced himself as Dr. El-Sheikh. He was the head of the department, and it just so happened he would be Esther's primary care physician. He was not a young, goofy guy that I would have imagined for children's oncology. Rather, he was fifty-something with hearing aids and a slight stoop. His Middle-Eastern face was stoic but not unkind. He spoke briskly, explaining things clearly: business first.

Frankly, I was appreciative of that. If he had pussyfooted, I would have been irritated. If he had sat next to us, sympathetically putting his arm around us, the tears in my eyes would have overflowed, and all reason would have gone out the window.

Looking at the percentage of "blasts" in the blood from the tests we had done a few days prior, he was fairly certain: "There is a very strong chance your daughter has leukemia," he said. A bone marrow biopsy would confirm this diagnosis, and a lumbar puncture would ascertain how far it had spread.

Specifics would have to wait on further testing, but what she likely had is B-cell acute lymphoblastic leukemia (ALL). And it had an 85–95 percent cure rate.

I breathed a little easier—but not much. It was too easy to assume my child would be that one in ten. But that voice in the back of my head also said, *Maybe she doesn't have it. This nightmare could be over in a few days. That would be good. I've learned some valuable lessons, at minimal disruption and trauma to my child. We can go home more thankful. I can get behind this scenario.*

***

That was, however, not our story. At the time everything initially unfolded, it was easy to believe that a quick reprieve from everything would be good. We would grow in our faith; some friends and medical professionals would witness us standing strong despite the appearance of difficulties. And best yet, we would get to remain comfortable.

We love comfort. And I mean "we" as a family as well as "we" the human race. It's always easy to believe that the comfortable way is the best way. But that isn't the case. Being out of your comfort zone stretches and molds you and brings out the best and worst parts of yourself. And that is certainly what happened (and continues to happen) as we travel down this road. The news we got was not *good*. But we had peace in our hearts in the truth that *God is good*, even when our circumstances are not.

***

As we got situated in what would become our home away from home, I finally settled down to sleep in an uncomfortable green recliner, my little person nestled in my arms. She had been issued a crib that looked like a plastic cage, which I had immediately rejected. Even had it not looked so threatening, I knew my tiny co-sleeper would scream all night should I try to lay her in it. A bed was denied to us on the tenuous grounds of "safe sleep," so I opted to have her sleep on me in a chair all night under the guise of "breastfeeding." I made (and kept) a pact with myself to be awake every time the nurse came in that night (that's once an hour, for those of you keeping score). I was afraid of being told to put her in the crib and watching the horrifying situation become unbearable.

Tubes and wires coming off of this tiny person tangled around the two of us, further securing us as one entity. The profoundness of our connection only increased from that night.

A horrible green recliner is an unlikely cocoon. But it began my transformation into a cancer baby mama.

And it gave me back trouble.

"

Oct 16

The biopsy this morning went smoothly and confirmed that Esther has leukemia. It is ALL, which is not the worst type to have.

Tomorrow afternoon, Esther will be in the OR again, to (1) install a central line, through which medications can be more easily administered, (2) administer a first dose of chemotherapy, and

(3) do a lumbar puncture, which will help determine how far the cancer has spread.

We will likely be in the hospital 4–7 days after tomorrow.

Esther has mostly had a happy day. She was very excited to see Grandma and Grandpa! They raised her spirits and kept her busy.

Ways to pray:

1. Pray for the lumbar puncture to be good, for no cancer to be found in the spinal fluid.
2. Pray for continued good spirits from Esther. Pray she can play and be a baby.
3. Pray that we get good sleep, all of us. A hospital is a good place to treat cancer, but a very, very bad place to get a good night's sleep.
4. For God to be glorified.

Things to know:

1. Chemotherapy lowers your immune system. We will not be keeping Esther in a bubble, but please know if she gets a fever, she gets admitted to the hospital. So don't kiss those kissable cheeks, and don't come to our parties if you're sick, please.
2. We have felt your prayers. Oh my goodness, the overwhelming support. What a blessing each of you is. And your friends you've asked to pray. We know we are well covered in prayer. It is our #1 answer when people ask what they can do: PRAY. Our God is a good God who listens to our prayers.

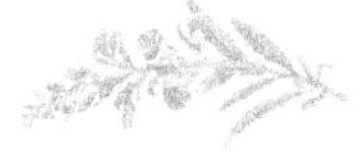

”

Dear Tired Parent

My dad is (or who I unbiasedly consider) the leading authority in wisdom. In the hospital, when we started meeting people, he would say, "Glad to meet you. Sorry you're here."

So, in that vein: Glad to meet you, sorry you're here. Wouldn't it be great if my book was allowed to grow moldy and dusty from disuse? Quietly slumbering in some forgotten corner of the library. Not because my writing was abhorrent, but because pediatric cancer had ceased to be a problem.

I suppose I can still hope for that. Big goals.

We probably won't meet in the halls of the hospital, because unfortunately, this pediatric cancer epidemic is not limited to one hospital, or even country. We're spread far and wide while we're being spread thin and ragged. But we stand together, and if we do ever meet in person, I can almost guarantee that we'll be immediate kindred spirits—as a certain Anne Shirley would be apt to say.

Love,

Sleepless in Ohio

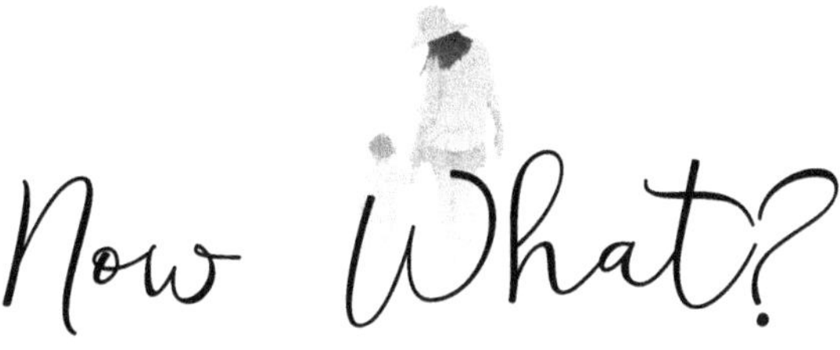

Now What?

Over the course of the next week, the dust started to settle, and we began to understand the ins and outs of our new normal.

Practically speaking, it was a lot to process. An incredible amount of information had been imparted to us by so many people, and trying to absorb it was hard enough on its own—never mind the emotional stress. We were learning about an illness that we had known only the most surface-level details. Did you know *chemo* is a generic term for dozens of varieties of this medical toxin? I didn't. We were told it would be a two-to-three-year treatment plan, which was a mind-boggling amount of time when you consider it was more than twice Esther's age at the time of diagnosis.

Leukemia protocols are generally preset, based on years of research and your child's specific subset of the disease. Other cancers have their own standards for treatment, sometimes tailor-made for a specific child. Your child also may be issued a risk level—i.e., standard, high risk, etc.—which will further determine the course of treatment. A series of time chunks, or cycles, make up the enormous calendar that is the foreseeable duration of the treatment. These cycles are generally one or two months, and our care team did not give specific details on more than the current cycle unless specifically asked.

At first it was frustrating to me that I was not getting information in advance. I am a planner, and I like to see things nice and neat on a calendar. Unfortunately, cancer is not *nice* or *neat*. Things change, treatments can be delayed, and ultimately, seeing the specifics of just one month at a time can be overwhelming. I think our care team realized this and spoon-fed families just one bite at a time. It seems manageable to do one task in a sea of undone chores, but sometimes the whole list can be daunting.

I once made the mistake of requesting several months at once, and our wonderful "nurse navigator" reluctantly supplied it to me. It was depressing. What gets you through a cycle of treatment is knowing that you will have that much more behind you—and maybe the promise that the next cycle will be easier.

No, it's never really easier. Every cycle is different, but it all kind of stinks.

The exception to this rule was the first month of treatment. It was undoubtedly the worst month of my and my husband's life. That's probably also true for my parents. And definitely true for Esther.

***

There is an automatic hand sanitizer dispenser outside every room in the hospital. After just a day, Esther started crying the moment she heard the noise outside our closed door. It meant someone was going to come in.

A plethora of people came into our room throughout the day. Doctors, nurses, assistants, cleaning staff, food staff, volunteers, and other medical specialists came in and out like we had a revolving door. And with every person, Esther cried. She cried especially when she began to recognize that all the nurses wore blue scrubs. I remember making a dreary prediction that blue would never be her favorite color.

With every person, we got new information. And it was like being a fully saturated sponge, having a trickle of water constantly trying to fill it up. And not to be dramatic, but despite my efforts, the leftover water oozed down my face.

A lady named Nancy was our "nurse navigator," a position I assume they assign based on organization and personability. For quite a while, hers was the only name I knew; everybody else was lost in a sea of nondescript blue scrubs and face masks. It was Nancy who sat down with us and went through a big, friendly binder, full of lovely charts and illustrations. The title was something like, "So your child has B-cell ALL. Now what?"

If my phone call from Esther's pediatrician was me being pushed out of a moving aircraft, this presentation was being shown where the parachute pull was. I was still falling, but not quite so out of control.

***

On one of the first few days we were admitted, Esther had a surgery to install a port under her skin in her chest. The purpose of this port was manifold: to ensure a perfect "stick" every time she needed an IV or blood draw; also, a chest port is necessary for chemo, as the fluid will wreck the smaller peripheral veins, especially in someone so small as Esther.

When talking about the port to everyone—staff, other parents, etc.—they were of one voice. "Oh, it's great! You're going to *love* the port."

I'm going to what, *now?* I'd think, while smiling politely. I'm going to adore and cherish this foreign piece of medical equipment in my tiny baby? This constant reminder of what she's living? I take her home and get to see a gash of a scar on her perfect baby skin, a hard lump just below it, where they slipped in a plastic doughnut to help administer chemotherapy. I don't get to forget about cancer even at home, when my tiny one is splashing around in the tub? Are naked baby bodies not sacred?

No. I could not summon positive feelings about this.

When they did the surgery for Esther's port, as with all procedures under anesthesia, she was required to be "NPO" for a certain amount of time beforehand. Real food was cut off first, and then breast milk, four hours before the scheduled procedure.

This was a serious problem for us. Not only was it a hunger issue, but Esther is a firm supporter of the theory that nursing heals everything—protects her from all. During this terrifying time in her small life, she sought frequent refuge at my breast, the safe place where bad things could not touch her. I frequently thank God for her being able to reap the breastfeeding benefits so thoroughly. Having this escape and respite saved her a lot of emotional trauma and kept her fed when she otherwise would have just gone hungry.

NPO is a Latin term (as are many medical ones): "Nil per os," or "nothing by mouth." Aspiration can be a risk when sedated—the chance of breathing something through the trachea other than air. Medical professionals want to keep vomit out of the equation when they're already doing something serious and complicated. Solid foods are restricted eight hours before a procedure. Breastmilk four hours. Clear liquids two hours.

Unfortunately, the time of her surgery kept getting pushed back, and four hours stretched to six or seven. The earlier offers of a breast pump—something I'd scoffed needing for maybe five or six hours—began to sound quite appealing, as I became acutely uncomfortable.

They brought a breast pump down from the NICU for me, and I laughed when I took a close look at what I'd produced. White, of course, but recognizably tinged with green.

"That's cancer-fighting boob juice," I confided to my husband. And then to about twenty of my closest girlfriends.

I do not remember what Esther got in the way of chemo on "day one" of treatment. I just remember thinking, *This is it*. I watched as the fluid descended from the IV bag into her tiny, perfect body. The horror of having to poison my child to heal her is a reality that will likely haunt me for the rest of my life.

"

Oct 17

The news is good. Esther definitely has just the "average risk" diagnosis that was originally put to her: ALL leukemia. No cancer was found in the spinal tap, praise God.

Even going smoothly, this will be a 2.5-year journey. Today is "Day 1." We will be in the hospital 5–6 more days and then back at least once a week for the first month. At that point, the hope is that the cancer is in "remission," and we will continue our weekly treatments to really knock it out. But that's for the future.

Chemo starts today, so we would ask for prayers for limited to no side effects and for the doctors to have wisdom in what they do for them (and in all things). Also, the risk of infection is ever-looming; we pray for no fevers or complications.

Right now, our primary prayer request (outside of good health and God's glory being known) is for Esther's emotional wellbeing. She is very physically drained today, and her fear of the nursing staff is intensified because of this. It's very hard to watch. It's also difficult to give her a rest from everything; our door is constantly opening and closing. The staff is great—it's just hard being at a hospital. They aren't made for resting. Babies need sleep and play and to feel safe.

Your prayers continue to lift us up, and we feel the Father near to us.

"

For all you fellow nerds who have seen the original *Star Trek* movie with the whale, I resonate strongly with Dr. McCoy as he observes twentieth century medicine and darkly calls it "the Spanish Inquisition."

(I knock it a lot, but at the end of the day, the chemo is healing my child. So I can't complain too loudly. Just a little loudly.)

The other thing that happened on "day one" was an assortment of oral medications. Which was an interesting feat of creativity for us as parents. How do you make a one year old take four medicines and a mouthwash without making her so mad that she throws them all up? With great difficulty, we discovered.

But we made it work. One at a time. We eased them into her mouth. Walked her around. She kicked and screamed. But by waiting twenty minutes between each one, we ensured that she didn't get angry enough to throw it up. And if she did, we'd only have to redo one and not the whole lot of them.

***

On "day four" of her treatment, Esther received a nasty little chemo called Pegaspargase. This chemo stays in the system for a month and is the most likely of all the chemos to cause an allergic reaction—5 percent of all recipients have some kind of serious reaction. An epi pen on hand, she was infused. And she made it through the next few days without incident, so it was determined that she was not likely to react.

"

Oct 20

Tomorrow Esther is getting the "day four" chemo treatment, which is a medication she has not had before. It is the one that most commonly elicits an allergic reaction, which is why we have to wait to cross this hurdle before we can go home. Assuming all goes well with it, we can go home Monday. Please be praying for this!

"

"But watch her for anything unusual," they warned. In fact, we were sent home with a full contingency of "just in case" instructions, along with many large paper bags of frightening prescription drugs. Some were her leukemia meds, and a lot were her side effect meds. One for nausea *without* vomiting. One for nausea *with* vomiting. One for acid reflux that the steroid gives her. And on and on. And very specific instructions for if she sprouted a fever.

If it's between 100.5 and 100.9, try again in an hour.

Bring her in if it's not better.

If it's 101 or more, she comes in—no debate.

They don't play around with the cancer kids, especially when so many fevers *could* be related to meds or the port. Everything is about being cautious. Playing it safe.

***

Turning the situation around and looking at things through a lens of thankfulness is sometimes very difficult. But it is essential. I saw these daunting medications and chemos and instructions, and I was overwhelmed. But the doctors weren't (and God certainly wasn't). Years of research have led to the current course of treatment, and the results speak for themselves. Pediatric leukemia "cure" statistics have increased dramatically in just a few decades. I know that treatment is always evolving, always improving. The system is complicated because it is being constantly honed. And I am thankful for the bright minds that brought us here and for all the medical professionals who are furthering leukemia cure successes.

"I'm just a graphic designer," I told (wonderful, irreplaceable) nurses when they got medi-geeky with their verbiage. When I consider all the years of education and hard work that go into the care of my child, I am humbled and thankful. And sometimes that's enough to get me through another day.

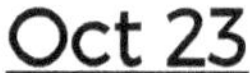

Oct 23

It's been a slow day at home. Esther is clearly glad to be home, but spent the day close to me, wanting to nurse a LOT, acting like she didn't feel very well. Lots of napping and laying on her mama.

She ate a very solid amount of cheese today, and bits and pieces of other things—but that mozzarella was just hitting the spot!

Medicine is displeasing, but despite retching, nothing got thrown up.

Tomorrow we have a quick blood draw at the Beavercreek satellite office, and then on Thursday there's a lumbar puncture (under general anesthesia) and her "day eight" chemo treatment. It'll be a long day, but outpatient.

Beloved and Overwhelmed Caregiver,

I know it seems hard now. It'll stay that way. Just kidding. Sometimes it will be worse.

But a lot of the time, it will seem manageable, and dare I say, even easy? Your friends will talk about taking their kid to soccer practice after school, and you will unironically equate it to your hospital extracurricular activities.

Of course, you'll have strange out-of-body experiences where you look down on yourself and wonder how you're coping with a child in intense treatment for a potentially fatal disease. Is it even mentally healthy to be so used to this horrifying alternate universe? I know we live in a time where mental health is being prioritized above its former status (this is good), so I won't dare to try to be a professional about this. I seem to recall not taking my psychology class in high school seriously anyways.

But this mom who's in the trenches tends to think normalizing your experiences is healthy. As much as you can. If you did nothing but freak out and spend life on high alert, that would appear to be unhealthy. And worse, it would probably cause stress wrinkles. We're trying to make it through this thing young and beautiful, am I right?

But seriously, please don't be afraid to seek help for yourself if you need it. On an airplane, they tell you to put your own oxygen mask on before helping others. So, for the love of everything, please be sure to take care of your precious self. You are so important. And if that doesn't speak to you, know you're going to be a hundred times better as a caregiver if you're not constantly in a state of high stress.

Love,

A mom who's afraid to look too closely at her roots because she suspects she's developing gray hairs

Steroid Cheeks

"

Oct 25

Today has been rough. Esther knows the hospital now and was antsy from the moment we stepped onto the Hem/Onc floor. Her anxiety only increased with every interaction with medical professionals, no matter how innocuous. I did a lot of walking her myself, as nothing and no one else would do. She was beside herself by the end of the day.

Lots of "hurry up and wait" happened, and we ended up being at the hospital from about 8 a.m.–2 p.m., doing her chemo and lumbar puncture. She did "well" with everything.

The only new medical information of significance is that they have uncovered one genetic abnormality. They have to do more genetic sequencing on it to see if it's potentially concerning. But it's one of those things there isn't perfectly definitive research on, so much of the process will be "wait and see."

Please be in prayer that this genetic information would not be a hinderance to her cure. Please also pray that she would "deprogram" from the hospital quickly. Even at home these last few days, she's not been her happy, goofy self most of the time. It's hard to watch.

Praise God, though: her numbers are good. As far as we can see now, the treatment is doing its job. November 14 is the day of her next lumbar puncture, and the end of this first month. From there, we'll be able to determine the next step.

If all goes well, we won't go back to the hospital until the next chemo infusion in a week.

Thank you again for your prayers, likes, kind words, etc. We read every comment and are encouraged. And your prayers are felt. God is near to us.

"

It was a foregone conclusion that the chemo would be rough. But we were unprepared for the steroids.

Esther took steroids by mouth every day, twice a day for a month—the first month of treatment. Like her other medications, she screamed through them. But the doctors told us that it really was a pretty nasty taste. And the side effects were worse. Oh, the side effects.

We were told that steroids can rob kids of energy. They get mood swings and can have uncontrollable rage and emotion. It'll make them feel like they have the flu. And they'll be hungry. A friend who went through parenting a toddler with leukemia a dozen years ago laughed, telling us stories about how her little boy would wake her up at three in the morning, demanding a full meal—which she, of course, cooked. Because that's what moms do. So I was prepared for that.

What I was not prepared for, however, was watching my vibrant, active toddler slowly become inert. The walking, which had returned briefly, quickly went by the wayside. And the crawling soon after. I watched my baby become replaced by a slow, tired version of herself, only interested in eating and nursing. Toys that she once loved, she lost interest in, immediately fussing and demanding to be returned to her mama milk. Her days were overtaken by the desire to sleep—awake long enough to chow down in her high chair, then nurse back to sleep.

> **Oct 31**
>
> The last few days have been sleepy days for Esther. We've relaxed at home mostly, eaten a lot of Cheerios and cheese, and napped lots. Sleep is good for healing little bodies!
>
> Please be in prayer for tomorrow. It's just a normal chemo infusion at 8:30 a.m., but I suspect it will be traumatic and scary for Esther to be back at the hospital. A shelf of medications with side effects are probably to blame for Esther's somber week, but I'd guess she's processing many experiences in her baby brain. It's a lot of disturbing things that have happened in the last few weeks, which are at odds with the 100% safe and peaceful life she's lived up til now. I pray she will be resilient and smiling again soon.
>
> (Below: Icing face yesterday, courtesy of Becky (a close family friend). We're trying to gain back that weight we lost at the hospital! Do pray for that also.)

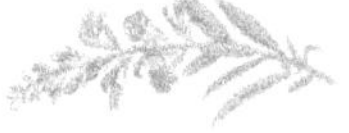

My baby girl quickly got the promised "steroid cheeks," which everybody commented on and appeared to love. And yes, I love a chubby faced baby. *But this face wasn't my baby's anymore.* I looked into her face and had a hard time finding my child. Every mother spends a countless amount of time staring into the face of her perfect baby, knowing every square millimeter, memorizing the curves and rolls, getting to understand the subtleties of expressions and emotions.

The face I had gazed at for countless hours over the past year had changed. And not just physically. You could see the tiredness and dullness in her eyes; it was like she was living in a fog. I felt like I was betraying my child to not be able to recognize her as the same little girl. But in reality, illness changes people—physically, mentally, emotionally. I was lucky enough to have her face back to normal a few months later, but the hair would be gone at that point. And I'll never know what to blame on the cancer process in the future; what trauma can I lay at its feet, and what was a natural failing in her nature?

> **Oct 29**
>
> Thank you all for praying. We're still not 100% (as evidenced by the non-smiling photograph below), but Esther is beginning to get back to herself. She was actually giggly right before bed, and I thought my heart would burst.
>
> Medicine taking was tolerated. In addition to the normal ones, she got a dose of anti-nausea medicine today, because I felt like it would help. She laid on me a fair amount but did some toddling and mischief making. Good quantities of Chick-fil-A and spaghetti were consumed at mealtimes.
>
> A pretty nice day.

Of course, it's possible she's picked up strength and bravery too. It's not all bad. And we can't go backwards; we move on and are thankful for the graces that rise out of the situation.

As the weeks dragged on, I found myself watching the calendar, marking days mentally that we had left before the steroids ended. Anything had to be better than this. Anything.

***

We had a week left on the steroids when I noticed my child beginning to turn yellow. Never a good sign. One day, it was so subtle that it didn't even register in my consciousness. The next day, I took note and called in to the hospital. I talked to Dr. C, another doctor on the team, who had me explain in great detail what I was seeing, and he determined that it was fine until the next day when Esther had scheduled chemo.

"

Nov 7

After all our rough emotions the last couple days, it was good to go to church and watch my child eat truly baffling quantities of pasta.

Thank you all (again) for your prayers and kind words! As I hit "like" on each of your comments, know that's my way of hugging you close and thanking you deeply. Your words often make me cry (in a good way!) and I wish I had the time to respond meaningfully to each of you.

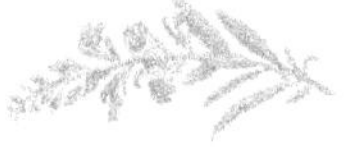

"

The next day, she was clearly jaundiced. At the hospital, the team took one look at her before preparing for admission.

When we arrived at the room, there was a bed instead of a crib.

"Oh, I'm sorry, did you want a crib?" asked the patient care associate (PCA).

"No," I replied, smiling broadly. "This is just fine." Small graces and big graces pepper our cancer experience. I tend to call this one a big grace.

"

Nov 8

Update from the hospital!

We came in for Esther's chemo infusion, but of course, life is not straightforward! She's had a bit of jaundice creeping in over the last 36 hours (if you saw me looking distracted yesterday, there's the reason!), and the liver blood numbers are off enough that the chemo treatment will be delayed. We're also being held overnight for "observation," as it's faster and simpler to do some of the necessary testing if she's inpatient. She's got a lot of chemicals going into her body (it's a lot for her liver to handle) so that's the layman's explanation and likely answer. Tests will reveal more specific ways her treatment can be modified for her body to process things better.

Her hemoglobin numbers were also low, so she's currently in the middle of a transfusion. This will hopefully raise her energy level just a bit too (she's already pinker!). She's being given O-, since there is no B- in the blood bank. So far, so good! (They always seem to be low on B- blood, so if that's you, feel free to come donate! It cannot be earmarked for a specific patient, but it's helpful for someone and could end up being used for Esther).

Her other blood numbers were good. And she did eat a couple french fries when we arrived, but I'm not sure how interested she's going to be in table food while we're here.

Her bone marrow biopsy should still happen on schedule on Wednesday.

Later, a nurse appeared to deliver a lecture by rote on "safe sleep." I nodded politely and proceeded to spend the next ten days in bed with my tiny, sick child.

Time passes strangely at the hospital. I often compare it to being on a cross-globe flight. It feels like you've been there forever and like the world outside is passing at a different rate. Like you're not part of the world anymore. You're tired and bored, but there's nothing to do but wait. And it feels like it will never end. Einstein's theory of relativity is proven on airplanes and in hospitals.

Six days of steroids left. The doctors ran countless tests to ensure they knew what the cause of the jaundice was. One of these was a liver ultrasound, and my baby was once again denied nursing for hours on end. I walked her endlessly through the halls in her carrier as we waited it out. Medicines were added to the regimen in an effort to bring down bilirubin levels.

Nov 8

Today went well.

Esther had an ultrasound of her liver and other neighboring organs, so she had to forgo food and breast milk for four hours preceding that (which is a dangerous thing to do to a baby with steroid-fueled hunger and rage). I walked the hallways a lot with her in a carrier.

However, 50+ images later, she was allowed to nurse and eat (some hot dog being the food of choice), and that combined with the blood transfusion earlier made for a semi-perky baby. Then the not napping all day caught up with her, and she crashed hard.

But we are (drumroll please) on a BED. That's right, a BED! I'm thrilled. I don't know if it's a fluke or if I was just the right level of confident, but I'm not questioning it. (For those of you who don't know, we co-sleep at home, and there's 0% chance of her sleeping in a hospital crib. When we were here for a week, I slept in an uncomfortable recliner, holding her.)

Praise God for beds. Pray no one tries to enforce any "rules."

Pray her test results are good, and solutions would be simple.

Pray for wisdom from doctors and staff.

Pray God would be glorified.

”

Five days of steroids left. Even more tests. A consulting GI doctor requested an untainted urine sample, which means a quick catheterization. My heart was in my throat in the time leading up to the test, and my eyes burned with tears as they pinned my baby down and caused her pain that she couldn't rationalize. Esther slept for fifteen minutes at a time, between knocks on our door. Sanity was quickly escaping me.

Nov 9

It's been a day of adventures. Lots of tests, lots of pain and discomfort, and scary things for baby. But the doctors are trying to rule things out and get to the bottom of this quickly.

Liver numbers are still all over the place. Various fluids and medications and blood products have been administered . . . I've honestly lost track. For the most part, though, they're trying to give her as little as possible to give the liver a rest. But a lot has happened regardless.

And we have been moved to the PICU, not necessarily because Esther is critical but because she could easily become so. Also, the nurse ratio is much lower on this floor, and there is a doctor ALWAYS on the floor, even at night. Our Hem/Onc doctors felt better about her being moved here, and we trust them.

Mostly, right now, it's a lot of hurry up and wait. We're waiting on test results to point our direction and nudging Esther's body along to heal in the meantime.

My parents will be arriving late tomorrow afternoon to take on some of the physical and emotional burden with us.

(More than ever, it is very important that Esther not be exposed to germs!! So please bear this in mind if you are thinking of visiting.)

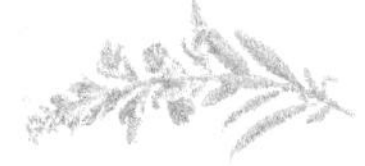

Four days of steroids left. We were upstairs in the PICU, as of last night. Everybody who's anybody in Hem/Onc has spent some time on the PICU floor. The doctors assured me it was just a precaution, and Esther was stable.

They brought in a massive machine that purified the air and sounded like an airplane engine. Apparently the PICU air is not filtered quite so thoroughly as the Hem/Onc air.

Three days of steroids left. We lived for the poops my child made, as every passing load meant her body was passing the trouble. My parents came to visit again and kept us alive with their morale-boosting conversation and quiet knack of knowing just the right things to do.

"

Nov 10

Today was a good day of rest. Yes, there were five thousand oral medications, and yes, Esther is plugged into so many cords and wires that she probably qualifies as bionic—but things were as relaxed as they could be. Esther was able to nap, doze, nurse, eat, and yes, fill her diaper. Which are all things that Mom, Dad, and the medical team agree she needs.

She could be better at eating table food, but we're not complaining about what we've got. It's definitely the best she's ever done in the hospital.

I will spare you the poop details, even though I'm so glad I could gush about it. Suffice it to say, it was the most impressive #2 she's ever made. Exactly what her system needed (and continues to need).

Also, my parents arrived! They're always my heroes.

Pray for her cycle of eating and voiding to continue. It may take a few days, but she needs to be doing these things for her body to repair.

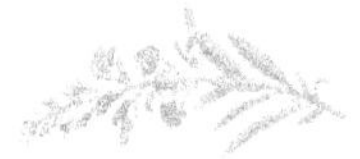

"

Two days of steroids left. Every employee at this hospital had now seen at least one of my boobs. Esther spent so much time on me, awake or asleep, that I was constantly exposed. And the endless procession of people through our door must have meant that all have seen what I'd prefer to keep private. But at this point, I didn't even care.

"

Nov 13

Every day, I count down how many doses of steroids are left. The amount of energy Esther has just dwindles a bit more with every dose. Thursday morning will be the final one for now. In theory, she should begin to perk up again slowly after the sequence ends.

All her liver numbers are improving, with one exception, and she is much less yellow. The bilirubin has dropped from the 13/14 range to the 6/7 range in one fell swoop, praise God. (Normal is below 1.) Her triglycerides have been rising this whole time, and they're starting to get into the realm where we begin to worry about pancreatitis. But for now, we just hope and pray for her body to continue to improve and the numbers to drop on their own.

Tomorrow is officially the procedure day. At 6 a.m., Esther must go off solid foods, and at 8 a.m. she's cut off from her favorite food source (i.e., me). The OR is scheduled for 12 p.m.

Esther will have a lumbar puncture. During this, she will have spinal chemo. Esther will also have her bone marrow biopsy, which will determine if she is in remission (we will not have the results of this for several days). And while she's under sedation, they will also give her an NG feeding tube (tube in the nose, straight to the stomach). Her protein has been low as a result of this whole ordeal, and this is the best way to get some supplemental nutrition in her. It's possible she will eventually go home with this tube.

And how about going home? It'll probably be at least the weekend, honestly. This liver process is just slow going.

Please pray for her liver, especially that one number, to improve further. Pray for her time without food to be easy and go quickly. We've had two of these sessions during this hospital stay, and they've been ugly. Please pray for her procedures to go well and for her to not be afraid at any point.

We covet your prayers in serious earnest. We pray for our daughter as often as we breathe, but it's easy to get caught up in the physical daily challenges. You are our prayer army.

One day of steroids left. Tomorrow morning would be the last dose. Esther had an NG tube placed during an LP procedure, much to my displeasure. Her weight had been dropping, despite the constant nursing and eating. I kept my sarcastic comments to myself. But seriously, she couldn't stay awake to eat because of the steroids, and the chemo made her sick. What do you expect?

Nov 14

This first photo below is marinara sauce, not something more scary! It has been the food of choice for the past few days. She's very passionate about this food right now; the folks in the kitchen probably laugh every time we order. We hide all kinds of protein sources in it!

This morning was pretty awful, but once we got her into the procedure room and sedated, things went smoothly. Esther had her LP, spinal chemo, bone marrow biopsy, and the NG feeding tube installed.

After the procedure, she was a bit dopey, but relatively happy. She nursed a bit and ate some (there's the photographic evidence!) and then we all napped for about an hour. When she woke up, she was limp but pretty perky for these days, so we played a bit.

She's a little grumpy and tired now (but eating again!); I'd guess she's feeling headachey from the procedures. Later tonight, they'll be giving her a feed through the NG tube, so hopefully that will go well. She's actually been gaining weight without it, and her protein was up a little this morning. So we are hopeful the team will not find it necessary to send us home with the tube in. It would be just one more thing to deal with.

The fringe benefit of the tube, though, is that her seven multiple-times-a-day oral medications can be given through the tube. This will make for a happier baby.

Speaking of medicine: only two more steroid doses left. Tonight and tomorrow. I'm dancing!

Also, they had people from a fancy salon going around giving out haircuts! Robert did not have time to partake, but I got a whirlwind twelve-minute haircut. Feeling light and breezy!

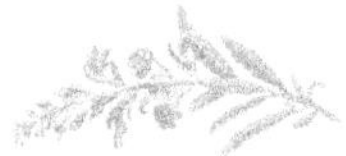

An NG (nasal gastrointestinal) tube is one which goes through the nose and down into the stomach. It is used for short-term feeding for someone who does not eat enough by mouth, or for administering medications to a reluctant subject. As to the former, Esther only ended up doing two nighttime feeds at the hospital, which seemed to upset her stomach, so mama bear told the team we were not going to do any more. The latter was a silver lining for us, as we didn't have to exorcise the medication demons for a full month (and after that, Esther got much better at taking her medicine).

An LP (lumbar puncture) is a procedure in which a needle is inserted between vertebrae near the base of the spine, to extract spinal fluid for tests or to remove fluid and insert medication. Part of Esther's protocol dictated frequent LPs to give her intrathecal chemotherapy. Adults are not generally put to sleep for this sort of procedure, but at our children's hospital, they sedate everyone for LPs.

The last dose of steroids was given one fine morning, amidst great cheering from the parents and grandparents. This was as low as we would get with this infernal medication.

***

I took stock of the situation. I saw how far we had fallen after we got pushed out of the airplane . . . .

Esther was barely sitting up. She could not sit on a soft surface unaided, and it was not just the roly-poly nature of her new, temporary body. Swaying gently and leaning into me to continue nursing was almost the extent of her motion, although she did sit in a high chair to eat.

I took videos of her sitting without leaning back to show her physical therapists. Whenever she had a PT session, she usually did not cooperate with their agenda. Crying through it, she would struggle on the floor limply, before giving up and screaming. It was disheartening and would leave a bad taste in Esther's mouth for the rest of the day. But the therapists were good and gave us simple activities to encourage those muscles to reactivate.

We were moving forward, though. Every step was absolutely in the right direction. The steroids, the "backbone of the treatment," had not felt like they were *forward*, but we knew they had been, and everything beyond them seemed less daunting.

***

November 20, 2018.

Remission.

The day Esther turned fourteen months, we got the news we had hoped to hear. Our sweet baby girl was in remission. God would be good if she had not achieved that. But we praised His grace towards us. And we took a deep breath and stepped bravely into the next two and a half years of treatment.

For Esther's particular brand of cancer, the care team aimed for remission after the first month of treatment—and usually achieved it. However, the additional treatment had been deemed necessary to minimize the chance of recurrence.

> **Nov 20**
>
> And we have remission!!! 0% on the cancer cells, and 0% on the genetic factor. Praising God every day, but especially today.
>
> More info later. Blood was collected to check her liver status. We'll hear back about that.
>
> The next round of treatment will not begin until next week. Whether she is treated as average risk or high risk depends on our doctor's consultation with some colleagues across the country. The genetic factor makes it a gray area. Pray for wisdom from them all, that the right choice will be made. Special prayers for our doctor, Dr. El-Sheikh, to make the right call.

Hey, Brave Mama,

I occasionally ask my nurses if I'm getting to be too annoying. I think the longer I'm in the "cancer mom" world, the more direct and (seemingly) bossy I tend to get. Or maybe I've just been reading too much Jane Austen lately and am expecting five delicate beat-around-the-bush questions to precede the actual meat of the matter.

Whatever the reality, nurses usually tell me they're glad I know what I want and that it's refreshing to have somebody who knows what's going on. So if you are in the wonderful position of knowing what's going on and what you want, please feel free to express that to everyone relevant. In a polite way though, please. We're not animals.

A mother's job is to advocate for her child. A mother of a sick child does that on a new level. A mother of a sick child who cannot communicate is performing some kind of psychic magic; it is a completely irreplaceable position to be in. There is nobody more able than you to explain how a little one is feeling. Don't worry that you're not qualified for this, friend. Because you are the expert in your field. (But the doctors have definitely had just a little training in oncology, so you should trust them quite a bit, medically speaking.)

Love,

The "Oh no, it's her again" Mom

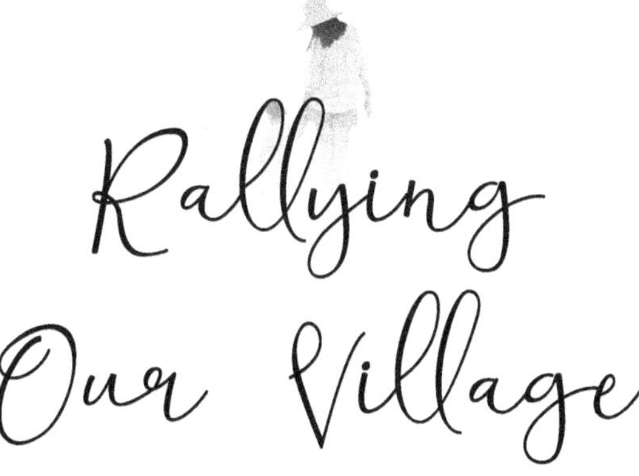

Rallying Our Village

> "
>
> **Dec 2**
>
> Esther has dealt pretty well with the chemo over the last few days. We've dosed her with anti-nausea meds a fair amount (every time she starts with the "uuurp" sounds), but it seems to be slackening off. Hopefully it was one of the Wednesday chemos causing this, and it's wearing off. She's been basically happy through it all though, even when I'm sure she's nauseated!
>
> Please pray for her weight to not drop and for her appetite to pick up. She's not been overly interested in table food since Wednesday.
>
> She has been a trooper about the nurses in our house the last few days too. She was sent home with her chest port accessed (tube out, ready to be hooked up) so she could receive a short IV chemo (ARA-C) on Thursday, Friday, and Saturday. Clearly it was mildly disturbing, having nurses in her house, but she still significantly charmed the two ladies we had—lots

of wrinkle-nosed grins. And yesterday when she was de-accessed (dressing pulled off, needle removed), Esther just sat and stared down the nurse placidly. It was impressive to all!

Just the once-a-day oral chemo alone for the next few days (it's a 14-day cycle right now, we're five days in). Please remember us in your prayers through this. We have to change her diaper every two hours when she's got chemo in her system, and for 48 hours after it's done. So these parents are not always well rested these days, especially Robert! He's our nighttime diaper changing hero. His superpowers include putting chemo gloves on in the dark and not yelling at me when I'm supremely unhelpful at 3 a.m.

Wednesday, we go back for a spinal chemo LP and the first of the four-day ARA-C again.

"

Getting Esther back to her physical baseline was an all-consuming task that almost seemed to overshadow the constant chemotherapy. It was something tangible we could strive for, whereas the cancer was a nebulous kind of foe, one we could not do much about as parents. But getting her walking again was a goal we could put our teeth into.

It took several months to get Esther back to just walking and even more time to get her to where she had been *before*. Even a year-plus later, she was still not physically where her peers were. But we thank God for progress and are grateful that her cognitive abilities and fine motor skills are not impaired. In fact, our daughter is quicker than many others to learn a new skill, and it is both amazing and a relief to see that.

Nov 29

A lot of people have asked, so I'll be a know-it-all about my newfound area of expertise: *So, what does remission mean for Esther?*

For a lot of cancers, "remission" means the treatment is done, or at least, drastically reduced. This is not the case with childhood leukemia. It also doesn't mean she is definitely cured, although we're definitely going in the right direction.

Esther still has 6–8 months of fairly intense treatment to get though, all the more intense now with her being on the "high risk" track of treatment. And then a further two years beyond that, maintenance treatment. And then after that, she will be regularly checked for recurrence. Probably for her whole life.

Doctors have just found over the years that this is the best way to fight the disease. Even though the cancer cells are not detectable right now, it doesn't mean they aren't there. If we stopped treatment now, the cancer would most likely come back quickly.

All that to say, we're over the moon about remission. It's a big deal. But it's not the end of the cancer.

And a short update: Yesterday was good. Really good. I guarantee God's hand in it. The only extended fussing was when they did that port access. She was not happy at some points, but never inconsolable, and usually happy. So, thank you for your prayers. So many thanks.

Today has been pretty good too. Some nausea—she woke up happy but giving some signs of an upset belly. And she threw up a bit before we could get the anti-nausea meds in her. But she's been doing some good playing and getting stronger physically.

She actually held a crawling position without any support and went backwards a bit!

The home care nurse came today and gave Esther her chemo. There was some anxiety from Esther about all the "hospital things" happening at home, but she did OK.

(The photo below is from Esther's lumbar puncture yesterday, which I was allowed to be in the room for. It was actually pretty cool to be there for! The doctor doing the procedure had a student he was explaining it to, so I got a free education. I told him I was good to perform the LP next time myself. He wasn't as amused by me as I am.)

”

Some people talk about the resilience of children, and it is referenced in many capacities. Orphans or foster children are called resilient. Kids who have suffered an illness, accident, or other trauma are lauded for their ability to "bounce back." And I think there is some truth in that, just as I think there is some truth in the opposing camp—those who hate when children are called "resilient."

Nobody suffers a trauma without scars, even children whose bodies are designed to grow and heal more quickly. I think kids just learn to survive and thrive around the scar tissue more effectively. As adults, it is our job to recognize their hurt and be sensitive to noticing what harm has come of trauma. And to help them thrive.

I don't know the long-term effects that will come out of Esther's cancer. Will she be easily frightened? Will she have separation anxiety? I don't know. All I can do is try to be ready to field it.

Dec 9

For the first time in many, many weeks, tonight this kid stood by the tub as I undressed her for bath time, instead of me holding her like a floppy infant. It's a tiny, huge milestone.

And tonight, she ate a decent dinner. Not sure it's indicative of future performance, or if it's a sign that her weight will be up, but it was good to see.

And Esther is acting like the spunky goofball that she is. What a joy!

Just a short post to tell you that prayer absolutely works, and our God is good and merciful. He has been giving us an abundance of grace-filled moments. Thank you for being faithful in prayer. Don't stop!

I'm not living my life sad. We do the treatments; it's just what we do right now. But sometimes it hits me. I look into her peaceful, sleeping face, and I notice that her eyelashes are falling out. This, on top of her very thin hair, makes a lump in my throat. *It shouldn't be like this.* Especially not for a barely one-year-old child.

"Other life" continues on in the midst of cancer. And it's easy to feel isolated from others. *How can they understand?* It's a constant battle, every day. Even small, normal things can be difficult or a reminder. We can't go swimming because her port sometimes remains accessed for a week. She can't walk over and get a book because she's feeling too bad. Dinner can't be normal because if she eats too much after chemo, she'll throw up.

But that's probably life. In our self-centered view, nobody understands exactly. Which is true, but most people in the world are "going through" something, whether it be illness of themselves or a loved one, death of someone close, or just a difficult life circumstance.

It's just another reminder to be kind to all and to check up on our friends.

"

Dec 13

Friends, it was such a good day. We were floating on a cloud of prayers. Esther was happy, she ate here and there, and she had a very long, restful nap. No throwing up. Just a brief bit of "urrrp!" when she woke up—which we headed off with medicine. Haven't needed to re-dose.

Tomorrow morning, Esther and I will head to Children's for an 8:30 a.m. infusion of Erwinia. Hopefully we'll be home around lunch time, where we get to greet Granny, Pop, and Uncle Ben.

Please pray for no side effects. Everybody dismissed the nausea as "definitely not the Erwinia," but I don't want to be the surprising exception, so I welcome your prayers. (If you're wondering, it was either an LP headache or just the combo of everything that day—it was a lot on a 22 lb. person!)

Also, please pray for the Walkers to wake up healthy and for smooth travels! We are so looking forward to their visit.

"

One tool that I found especially effective in aiding communication and prayer was social media. A few days into our original hospital stay, either Robert or myself dully observed that perhaps we should set up an update page for

Esther. So I, the photographer and writer, began using my giftings in a wholly unexpected way.

The first few posts were hard to write. It was difficult to grapple with the reality that my child had every right to a rallying slogan: "Esther Strong!", "Esther's Fight!", or some other heartening language. We settled on "Praying for Baby Esther," as it was descriptive but didn't give me a weird feeling in my stomach. Maybe an older kid would be strong or have a fight, but Esther doesn't even know what's going on. She's just living her life, not knowing anything is different. She's not a celebrity slogan on a T-shirt; she's one year old. (But we know a lot of strong fighters who have every right to the celebrity status!)

Pegaspargase (Peg) is a chemotherapy drug which boasts a notable percentage of extreme adverse reactions. Erwinia, or Erwinase, substitutes for when the Peg is deemed an unsafe risk. The core drug is the same, but the mixing agent makes this alternative more tolerable. Instead of remaining in the body for close to a month, it only stays in the system a few days. This translates to more doses of Erwinia when a patient would normally just need one of the Peg.

The praying part was what we coveted most. Feeling helpless brings you closer to the Lord, which is perhaps a reason why we shouldn't rely on miracles and be devastated when they don't happen. Sometimes we walk a hard road, but God walks with us. As do our many faithful friends.

Coming to our Facebook group during times of great distress was an enormous comfort. To have the support of a community at the tips of your fingers is not only a massive morale boost but is a prayer force to be reckoned with. As soon as I'd hit "enter" on a post, my heart would feel calmer. My breathing would steady. I would clean up vomit-soaked sheets and shower the chemo puke from my hair while my husband rocked a whimpering but more peaceful baby. In between these necessary ministrations, I would check up on the post. Every few moments there would be a new notification.

Praying for you.

Trusting in God to sustain you through this hard time. Hugs.

Prayers for peace, strength, and courage as you fight this battle. Remember, you don't fight alone.

March 28

Just wanted to write a brief note to say THANK YOU for praying for Esther's sleep! It's not every toddler mama who gets an army of people praying for her child's poor sleep habits. I am thankful to report that it was only the one night of sleeping weirdness. All has been normal since then—normal being Esther assuming the "H formation" in between Robert and me and nursing all night long, should she so choose. This is our life. We are happy.

Esther's tush rash is still there, but fading slowly with the stronger steroid cream. We are only to use it a week at a time, so I've stopped applying for now.

All is good here. Esther is back into her routines. Napping well. Playing happily (with the Mother Ship close by, naturally). Eating decently. Saying "NO!" a whole lot. Some of it is for the joy of communication, being understood. Some of it is toddler attitude . . . we're working on that!

And on and on. Every simple "praying" left me feeling cared for and loved, and the more involved commenting brought me to tears over my nocturnal sanitizing.

This fight is mainly yours, as a family, but don't be afraid to lean on others. Heck, they *want* to help. You just need to give your support group the information they need to help in a practical way.

Before we came home from our first hospital stay, we had given the word that it would be helpful for people to come to our house and sanitize, especially Esther's toys. A small army of ladies came and cleaned our house top to bottom. One of these ladies later gifted me with a huge stash of non-chemical cleaning supplies.

Esther loves Chick-fil-A. If she's going to eat at all, Chick-fil-A is top of her list. As soon as people found this out, we were swimming in CFA gift cards.

It's a long and sometimes lonely road, but don't make it lonelier than it needs to be. As with regular life, sometimes you have to do the reaching out in order to get results. And this isn't because people don't want to help or because they forget about you on purpose. It's because people aren't mind readers, and if you're putting on a brave face all the time, they don't know that you're in need of anything at all.

Chemotherapy essentially targets fast-growing cells (i.e., cancer cells). But other fast-growing cells include hair (which is why many patients are bald), mouth (which is why mouth care is an important factor in treatment), and white blood cells (which help your body fight other diseases). It is very important to keep an eye on your child's blood numbers to gauge their risk of falling ill. If numbers dip too low, it's important to be extra vigilant about hand washing, and potentially you'll want to keep your little one in a bubble, leaving home infrequently or not at all.

If you are breastfeeding your cancer baby, this is a bonus in absolutely every way. Not only does it help with nutrition and comfort, as I stated before, but it passes on so many antibodies to keep them healthy. If your little one is not nursing, or has aged past that, all is not lost! You just have to be an even bigger helicopter mom with the cleaning and personal sanitizing.

Gentle Cancer Parent Reader,

*I would encourage you, parent advocate, to have a social media page, email chain, detailed smoke signal, that you can update often. It feels self-centered and self-serving sometimes. It feels like a lot of work sometimes. Sometimes it makes you feel like a weird press agent, communicating with the world for your new celebrity. But it is an amazing tool. You get the most amazing gift—*PRAYER. *A group such as this gets you connected with those who want to know the ins and outs of treatment, without clogging up a personal account. You are not your child or your child's illness; it will take over your life for a time, but don't confuse yourself with either of those.*

(1) *Practically speaking, I would say only update when there is a reason. People have been very encouraging of my learning process with the page, saying they'd always rather hear more than less. "We want to know how to pray!" they tell me enthusiastically. And by golly, I want those sweet little old ladies and college friends and friends of my sister in a different state to know how to pray. But I also know human nature, and I don't want to tempt them to become tired of me or to let me become background noise. I want every post to be one read eagerly—with a joy to pray. My daughter deserves that.*

(Taking a different approach isn't wrong. I don't know that there's a right or wrong here. But this is my humble recommendation.)

So I post for several different reasons. If we have an appointment, I post a little blurb. If she has a blood test a few days prior to an appointment (in preparation), I post (once!) when I know the results, and if/when she will have an appointment. I also post if there is something that requires immediate prayer. Esther has been throwing up all day into the night and isn't able to sleep—that warrants a post. Sometimes it seems to add up. But you know what? People who follow the page want to know what's going on. They like reading the updates. They want to know how to pray. And if they don't want to read all about my kid's cancer? Well, that's OK. They don't have to follow the page.

(2) *And be honest. Be positive, be trusting of God, but be honest. It is not wrong to admit to feeling blue or defeated. That's human. And yes, you're super mom (or dad!), but you're also prone to those pesky human failings. Make sure you don't forget to give God all due credit, and remember to shine His goodness wherever you put metaphorical pen to paper. If you can't look for the goodness in your kid with cancer, it's going to be a dark time for you. So find it and share it with others.*

(3) *Stories of the everyday and of your friends in the hospital will color your narrative and bring your community closer. People are storytellers and story absorbers; it is how we grow and communicate. Don't underestimate the power of a good story.*

(4) *Take photos! And videos! Both for the public and for yourself. People want to see who they're praying for—and you'll be glad you take them for yourself. I had to force myself to take photos at first. I did not see how I would want to remember this. But time passes, and hospital life will grow less alien. It will be almost normal. And you'll want to look back on the beginning of the era and say, "Look how far we've come."*

(5) *Don't forget to use your newfound "fame" for good. Share about other friends in the Hem/Onc department (with abbreviated or code names—perhaps asking permission first). You don't know who is and isn't receiving prayer.*

I found someone who defined a blessing as something that brings you closer to God—something that points to Jesus. I am always hesitant to use the word blessing *because I think we overuse it in our western culture. But I guarantee, sharing God's goodness will always bless you and others.*

Love,

The Unexpected Documenter

The Fourth Floor: Our Other Address

This hospital gig was our new job: appointments at least once a week, sometimes more. Some days we literally spend 9–5 at the hospital, taking rush hour traffic in and out. We have learned a lot of information—unwilling students of the school of cancer. And it took some time for me to figure out our "normal" for this season. We were drowning after being pushed out of a plane, but after a few months, we broke the surface and began to tread water.

It was determined that the day four chemo, Pegaspargase (Peg), was what gave Esther liver failure. So she got the alternate chemo, Erwinase (also called Erwinia). Instead of getting one dose of the Peg, now Esther had to endure six doses of Erwinia in two weeks every time the protocol called for Peg—which ended up being seven more times.

> **Dec 12**
>
> Here we are! Left the house at 7 a.m., and she's had her Vincristine infusion. There has been happy playing and lots of mobility from the little explorer. The last half hour or so she's been cranky, but that's what happens when it's naptime!
>
> Currently EARLY for our LP (!!), and then we head back up to the infusion room for her Erwinia infusion. That's a one-hour infusion and a one-hour wait after.
>
> The Erwinia is the substitute chemo for the Peg, and the difference is that it stays in the system less time. So instead of one dose and done, we have to do six infusions over a two-week period, but it's less risky for her liver.
>
> (Update: Oh, and the NG tube is now out!!)

We were at the hospital *a lot*.

I tell people there are good and bad things about my cancer child being so young. On one hand, I don't have to explain the weight of the situation to her, and she doesn't know any different. She's pretty sure everyone goes to the hospital on the regular. But on the other hand, she can't tell me when she's feeling nauseated or is aching. I just have to rely on my mom instincts. These are sometimes stellar—and sometimes not.

Give yourself (and your child!) grace, fellow parents. This is uncharted territory.

When we go to the hospital, Esther usually regards it as an extension of her kingdom. This chick swaggers in and wanders the whole fourth floor. Everybody knows Esther. It took me a while to figure out that most kids don't spend 95 percent of their time out of their room. But Esther always wants to be out exploring, playing, and grinning coyly at admirers over her shoulder. At first I believed she just wanted to escape whatever room procedures happened in. But after a while, I think she truly came to revel in this giant playplace.

The Hem/Onc floor at Dayton Children's Hospital is essentially a giant square, one that you can walk all the way around through corridors. The first side is the waiting room. There are nondescript clinic rooms lining one wall, chemo/blood infusion rooms on the back wall, and inpatient rooms on the third. There are also a couple play rooms and parent rooms. This whole domain belongs to Esther. "Everything the light touches," we'd tell her solemnly.

And she ran things benevolently. Most days, she had a grin and a "no, no!" for just about anybody who crossed her path. Everybody always loved to admire her tiny flip flops, the bow on her bald head, or mostly just her sweet little face.

A lot of patients left their doors open, so it was an early exercise in training to tell her, "That room isn't yours. We don't go in rooms that aren't ours unless we are invited in." She learned this fairly quickly. She also learned that it was entirely acceptable to stand in open doorways and stare for an uncomfortable amount of time. As a toddler, who's going to yell at you for this? As the parent following the toddler around with an IV pole, it's easy for things to get awkward.

"Come on," I'd eventually say, nudging her tiny shopping cart with my foot. "Where are we going, Esther? Let's go!" And she'd take the hint after a while and rocket off with that plastic red and yellow kiddie cart, hollering like a wild woman. And I would race off behind her, pushing the IV pole and hoping for the best.

I'd compare this exercise to walking a dog, but since I really can't pull on the leash, it's like the dog is walking me. I suspect it is a favorite pastime of nurses to watch parents of toddlers chasing their tiny, rambunctious people, sweating.

Unfortunately, coming to the hospital is not all fun and games, as I've probably led you to believe by now. One thing Esther never did well with was being accessed, also known as having the needle put in her port. This process necessitated everybody in the room wearing masks and hats and holding the toddler down. The spot on her chest had to be cleaned and dried, and then the special needle was put in. A biopatch sticker was put on top, and then we were good to go—after having blood drawn and chemo connected, that is.

Esther does not like being held still, and I don't blame her. Having three or four adults looking down on you in pink face masks and lunch lady hats has to be not only terrifying but a violation of the Geneva Convention, I'm sure. So, there is screaming there.

And the Erwinia, the lovely replacement chemo for the liver failure chemo, turned out to be the only real nausea-inducing one for Esther. Everything else could be held under control with medication, but the Erwinia was stubborn for her. It kicked her butt every time. I tried every combination of medicine, eating, not eating, breastfeeding or lack thereof, and still her times of throwing up happened more often than not, and I couldn't pin anything to it.

All I could do was limit food somewhat and make sure she had an early appointment so she would be done with nausea before midnight. We'd do our patented limited mix of nausea medications as well.

"

Dec 14

Well, the good news is, we know what caused the vomiting. The bad news is, it is the Erwinia, the thing that it probably wasn't.

All the anti-nausea meds are being utilized. Please pray with us that today is not as bad as Wednesday. God has given us the ability to create these medicines, and has given us smart medical professionals. We pray they are being used to their best advantage for Esther.

The Erwinia is the substitute for the Peg. It's our only option. We just have to fight through the next few times with increased meds.

The other good news is, Robert's parents successfully are en route.

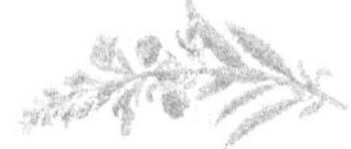

"

Having a child under two in the hospital is an interesting experience for many reasons, but there are some hospital policies and pharmaceutical rules about things for that age range that complicate it. For example, if you're over two, the official stance on co-sleeping is tolerated (hence why I was given a hard time our first stay).

Anti-nausea medicine comes in a million shapes and forms, but if you're under two, there are really just a couple of medication options. Benadryl did nothing for Esther on Erwinia except make her wake out of her drugged sleep to puke. An oral medication called Emend didn't hurt, so we'd throw it in the cocktail. A class/family of medications including Zofran and Kytril (different strengths) was our main weapon. We eventually changed our dosing frequency to help a little, but it was just such a problem chemo for her.

Prayer was very important in this particular cancer trial. On the nights when Esther was waking up to throw up, I'd cry out to God with tears streaming down my face. *Why does it have to threaten her sleep as well as her waking? It doesn't seem fair that she isn't allowed to indulge in rest, especially when it was the cancer medicine that was causing the discomfort, not the cancer.*

I am so thankful that Esther's cancer was likely caught early. But it confuses my subconscious that we're treating a disease that never gave her symptoms. To watch her struggle with horrible side effects feels like I'm betraying her, taking her to the hospital to poison her. I'm glad her logical thought is limited at this age, because she'd probably have some pretty irrational (and unfortunately rational) conclusions to draw.

It's a lot for a parent to process and work through, especially on a spiritual level. Being a follower of Christ, I'm always hopeful that this personal refining, squeezing process is one that points onlookers to Him. That is my prayer, alongside the omnipresent one for Esther's health. And it gives me joy to think that I am allowed to serve my Creator in a way that many people cannot.

By twisting my perspective just a little bit, I almost enjoy this unexpected mission field. It is a place to meet people I would have never otherwise encountered. The hospital is a great equalizer. We are all there for the same purpose.

Chemo precautions last for forty-eight hours after it is administered. If daily oral chemo is involved, it is ongoing until forty-eight hours after it ends. The idea is that chemo-laced bodily fluids are not good for anyone, especially the non-patients. If you get vomit or urine on you, you need to shower and wash it off as soon as possible.

Another fun aspect is the chemo diapers. Strict protocol is to change a diaper every two hours for someone on chemo (apparently chemo-infected pee causes diaper rash or something . . . who knew?). This was especially hard at night for us, when it went on for months at a time sometimes. Thankfully, we discovered a good rhythm and were able to go longer than two hours without adverse reactions. Knowing your child and learning their habits makes things easier in the cancer world and in the regular world.

And this purpose is a hard one, so I've given myself permission to have bad days. I'm allowed to cry at the unfairness and to need extra couch potato time instead of cleaning the bathrooms. I feel like it should not be as hard on me as it is. After all, I am not the one being repeatedly poisoned by my medication. But I am doing a full-time job of keeping my child alive. It is every parent's job to do this, but any child with special needs exacerbates this call. And if I didn't believe in a strong link between the physical and mental before, I do now. The sheer mental taxation of this stress wears you down. And that's OK and normal.

"

Dec 10

After a day of no signs of nausea and no throwing up, Esther woke up an hour after falling asleep to puke quite a lot.

This is after getting her anti-nausea meds every four hours today, which is as frequent as it can conceivably be.

Please pray for her to not throw up anymore. For her to sleep again soon and well. For her parents, who are so discouraged by this wretched chemo that our daughter has to take fifteen more times in the next two months.

There seems to be no means of fighting it and it is immensely disheartening.

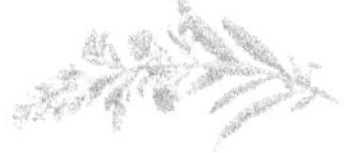

"

Dear One,

It never ends. This can be said of motherhood, fatherhood, or this joyful cancer merry-go-round you have accidentally boarded. Every time I think I have nothing more to say, I remember twelve things I wanted to share with you guys. The teeth enamel problems, which potentially spread from chemo side effects. Or maybe excessive (let's be conservative and call it fifteen times every twenty-four hours, many days) breastfeeding. The latter is probably some sort of psychological side effect of being repeatedly traumatized . . . so it comes back to cancer, and I get to tell our insurance provider that it's cancer related—so they should please cover it.

Or the dry skin patches, that I wonder if they are good, honest spots of genetically obtained eczema from her mostly perfect mother. I slather heavy duty lotion on them when they flare and wonder if it's a resurgence of that mysterious methotrexate rash.

I see parents further down the road who talk about learning disabilities and PTSD from their cancer kid—many years out of treatment. Fear spikes. Does it ever end?

If you are so fortunate to have a living, breathing child who at one point had cancer in their body, then no, it blessedly does not end. It continues. This is the price we choose to pay when we became parents. The stress and fear we daily need to offer up to God. Some days I'm better at that than others.

It stinks that life seems to be more generous to some than others and that we are not even allowed the small honor of taking 100 percent of the discomfort or handicaps from our children. But we do what we can. Because while our child still lives, we are parents. And if our child does not live, that title is not stripped from us.

Stay strong. It's not easy, but you are not alone.

Another Mother

Strangers Like Family

There's a saying among the pediatric cancer community: friends become like strangers, and strangers become friends. It's easy to feel isolated from people who don't fully grasp the enormity of your new normal—not because they don't want to, generally. It's the line between empathy and sympathy. You can imagine the crippling fear of your child having a potentially fatal diagnosis. As a mother, I think it's safe for me to say we've all imagined a hundred scenarios that end in tragedy for our child. But the difference is to step over that line and realize the concrete numbing horror of no escape from reality.

I feel that we were fortunate. Even though most of our friends did not have a similar frame of reference from their own lives, they wanted to understand. They wanted to help. For the most part, I think the abrupt change in our lives' path was a catalyst for deeper and more meaningful existing relationships.

And our cup of mercies and graces was added to. A few months into Esther's cancer treatment, I began to come out of the fog and started to notice individual people, instead of the faceless hospital entities and fellow purgatory sufferers. I came to realize that we had four main attending doctors. They rotated through the sections of the department, but they tried to always see "their" patients during a clinic visit.

It didn't always work out that we'd see Dr. El-Sheikh every time, so we did get to know the others: Dr. D, who always made a funny mouth sound to entertain kids (although it seemed to entertain the nurses more—they chuckled as they talked about his "kid noise"); Dr. C, who always seemed to get the brunt of my frantic "after hours" calls; and Dr. W, who engaged in Nerf wars with the teenage boys. If they shot him, he'd tell them the bullets would be returned later, in the manner of his choosing. And when "later" came, he could be seen roaming the halls with a very imposing Nerf gun.

There were two nurse practitioners, and both of them were gems of human beings, lingering in our room longer than strictly necessary to properly assess Esther's playtime ability. One of them cried when Esther said her name for the first time, and the other betrothed her toddler son to my toddler daughter.

I became besties with the nurses and nursing assistants, especially the infusion clinic ones. Most of them were ladies between 25–35, so it wasn't hard to feel comfortable with them. They were my *strange peer group*. You spend a lot of time with them in your room, hooking up chemo or taking vitals, so it's a foregone conclusion that you get to know them. I knew about T and her husband, ready to have kids, and I watched her go through the process of waiting followed by a joyful pregnancy. I was overjoyed for sweet E, for whom Esther always had a hug, when she married her fiancé. I had a memorable conversation with K about potty training her toddler. I heard about their pets and struggles and weird family members. I knew who worked what days and asked after them when they were missing. And when they didn't see us for a while, they were genuinely glad to have us there again. ("But we know you don't *want* to be here. Nobody *wants* to be here. But we are glad to see you! Esther is our favorite. Don't tell anybody.")

Secret's out.

The nurses were one of the reasons it was bearable—"it" encompassing all things relating to hospital-based cancer treatment that made us, as parents, want to sit down and cry in the hallways. It was even enjoyable sometimes. I called it my "expensive hotel spa" whenever we had to stay overnight—as many slushies as I could drink and unlimited stickers. Esther liked to put those on my bare skin, and it became my habit to forget they were there. This resulted in looks and smiles in and outside of the hospital and stinging red patches when I removed them.

I wasn't the only one sporting stickers or strange accessories on the Hem/Onc floor. When you're a parent of a cancer kid, you do anything and everything to make them happy. We met so many people.

It was a common sight to see Alicia chasing Braxton down the hallway: IV pole in one hand, his cup of water in the other hand, and the little man himself on a tricycle. Braxton is a force of nature and never ceased to make me chuckle. At two years old (about six months Esther's senior), he knew precisely what he was after—and he went for it. While Esther was a dainty fairy of a size, Braxton was solid—something no chemo could take. He had torn his accessed port tube multiple times by sheer force of being himself. Alicia was a down-to-earth mama bear, often claiming she was frightened or nervous, but all I saw was an unshakably strong woman, ready to fight alongside her son against his leukemia.

As I'd walk Esther and she'd stare in open doors, we met Ben, a young teenager with a sarcoma. His door was always open, his room filled with gifts and well wishes from a supportive community and family. He'd roll his eyes as his mom carefully taped up signs on the window, crafted lovingly by his little siblings. But his room was always full of positivity and joy. The first day we met them, when they were undoubtedly full of uncertainty and fear, Ben gave Esther all his balloons. She stopped by his room every circuit, gazing longingly at his trio of "babas," floating lazily in his room. One by one, he gave them to her. I cried in our room that night.

Tommy was another teenager, with a different type of leukemia: AML. Treatment was only four months, but it was very intense. He spent three out of four weeks admitted for that chunk of time. I had seen his mom, Joni, around quite a while before we met; she was distinct in her German Baptist garb. Despite our difference in age and life circumstances, we found we had a lot in common as we walked the halls together. She was a woman of strength who had gone through intensely difficult things even before this.

Henry, about a year older than Esther, had survived a brain tumor with incredible joy and grace. His smiles and kind words lit up the whole department. He and my little one played together a few times, and he would come up to me and say, "I hold you?" and climb into my lap. And my heart melted.

About the same age as Henry, Joey also rocked a high-risk leukemia diagnosis with Esther. He would always be pranking the nurses and finding sassy things to say. As a toddler should.

And we met Kelsey, who had diabetes along with her leukemia. Their family's house was destroyed by a tornado a few months after her cancer diagnosis. Despite all of this, their family was so full of love for everyone. I know her mom was stressed, but she'd always have a broad smile for us—and sometimes stuffed animals or balloons for Esther. Esther would wander away, smiling down maternally at her new toy.

"Say 'thank you!'" I'd remind her.

"Tankoo," she'd say softly to the toy, holding it close against her chest.

(I could mention more friends; we met so many kind people. Their strength was a unifying factor.)

Of course, I could also mention the hollow looks in our nurses' eyes some days. Days when it seemed like they had to work extra hard to smile for their patients they could still treat. And I could talk about one of our doctors, who spent several weeks on emotional autopilot. I wasn't brave enough to ask him the particulars, but heaven knows these medical professionals knowingly picked an impossible field to work in. You can save a lot of kids, but you can't save them all.

And forever imprinted in my mind is an empty hospital bed, tucked into a side hallway, waiting for somebody to have the time (or heart) to put it away. I had seen this particular bed, made remarkable by being a few notches in quality above the regular ones, in photos of fresh grieving and memorial the night before. That sweet boy didn't make it to double digits. I sit here writing tremulously with one hand, the other up against my face, holding myself together. The phrase, *I can't imagine,* is often applied by other parents in situations like this. Unfortunately, it's not hard for me (or you) to imagine the grief of his parents.

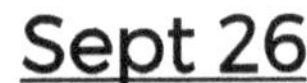

Sept 26

Just wanted to share a few photos from yesterday to illustrate that our long days at the hospital are full and varied. Yesterday Esther made and delivered cards to two inpatient friends, passed out on me before the LP because 6:30 a.m. is a wee bit early for her highness, and stuffed her face with pizza in a tiny red car. That's not including the medical shenanigans or lesser adventures (chatting with a favorite LP nurse, inopportune toddler poops, and birthday gifts). Also a bonus video of an audition to whatever reality singing TV show will take her.

She did well. Has continued to do well today. Did not have to do any anti-nausea meds today. (Which is a relief, since I'm already up to four syringes of meds a day at the moment. I'll have to briefly up it to five in a couple days.) She's been a bit tired but still happy and functional. Continues to impress her physical therapist (whom we saw today).

Sometimes I step back and look at what Esther goes through, and I'm amazed. What a wonderful tiny human she is. She handles things with more grace than many would (truly, including myself). And she's only two.

Please remember our friend K, who has been having unexplained seizures again. Pray they find a non-worrisome reason and can easily treat it.

And we are celebrating with our big friend, B. Many months ago, we met him and his family on their first stay in the hospital, full of uncertainty. And even so, all of their family radiated kindness and love. Esther made off with all B's balloons by the end of their stay.

Wednesday began his last planned chemo stay (of five days). It's not the end of worrying or side effects, but we are so, so glad, with their whole family, that he has reached this milestone. Please pray the cancer does not return.

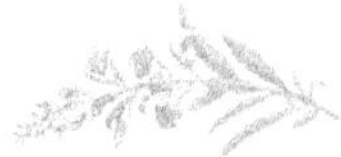

A two-year-old's birthday is always something of joy, but the anxiety-soaked relief of a momentous day is an emotion reserved for parents of medically complex children. Parents and children celebrate the day of diagnosis—after treatment ends. A kind of joyous spitting in the face of cancer, if you will. But every year when that day rolls around, it surfaces those feelings that originally happened on the dark day: fear, agony, crippling doubt. You have to celebrate, to trample those demons down. Heaven knows we need extra reasons to celebrate.

Birthdays and end-of-treatment anniversaries make more sense to the outside world, and we like those too. There are extra reasons to be thankful on birthdays. Nobody is guaranteed a certain number of birthdays, but a little kid with a cancer stamp on their file has been given an uphill battle on that front. As parents, we want to make each day count, especially the birthdays.

On her second birthday, Esther had a Tarzan themed party, with an incredible cake made by my wonderful friend and neighbor, Becky. We have all the Tarzan music lyrics memorized in this house. True to toddler form, Esther was incoherently inconsolable for two thirds of her party and had to be removed to an upstairs room for a significant chunk of time so she could recover from the indignity of friends playing with her old, pre-birthday toys. After, I vowed never again to throw her a party.

But what can I say? I'm incorrigible. It's very likely I will go back on this promise and live to regret it. All the while, in this fiasco of a celebration, I basked in the normalcy of a two-year-old who was feeling good enough to scream at her friends.

Brave Parent

I would encourage you to make friends. Meet people. Mentor and be mentored. Aim to get more from this experience than simply restored health, as important as that is. The difference you can make to a struggling parent in a simple five-minute conversation can be perspective altering for them. Or you.

Our hospital has digital displays outside each inpatient room—a screen bearing the first name of the occupant. If you've ever been on a prayer walk, you know that sometimes the hard part is knowing what to pray and who you're praying for. The beauty of prayer walking at the hospital is that you can pray for these kids and their families by name, and you probably can guess exactly what they need prayer for. And you can do it while jogging after an escaped toddler.

Remember their names. When you wake up in the night to listen to your small one breathe, go through the list of kids. Smother them in prayer. There's no such thing as too much prayer. Be bold in your requests, and remain faithful that God is able.

Love,

The Hospital Hallway Monitor

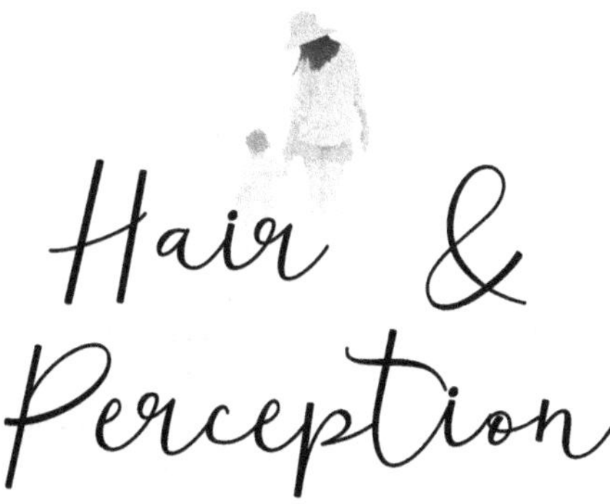

Hair & Perception

> **Nov 7**
>
> It's been a few hard days, and there are more ahead of us. The steroids have been leeching Esther's energy: she spends most of her time laying on top of us, either awake or asleep. There are maybe a few five-minute chunks in the day where she'll want to sit on the floor, and play. She hasn't even crawled in about a week. I haven't seen a smile crack her face in days: she's certainly feeling bad.
>
> And to cap it off, we've been finding little baby hairs everywhere. It's such a small thing, and we knew it was coming, but it's still hard.
>
> I say this not to depress you but to be real with you. We trust in God's sovereignty, but we're also human parents. This is undoubtedly the hardest experience of our lives. We couldn't do it without God, and we're glad we don't have to do it without you.

Please pray that God will give us all strength to get through this last (for now) week of steroids. Please pray Esther's IV chemo infusion tomorrow morning (10:30 appt.) would go smoothly, with minimal fear and discomfort for her. Please pray that everything else in her body is healthy and functioning as it should.

The big date we're all holding our breaths for is a week from today, Wednesday, November 14. Esther will have her regular IV chemo as well as be put under anesthesia for (1) a lumbar puncture to check that no cancer cells have made their way into her spinal fluid, (2) spinal chemo, and (3) a bone marrow biopsy to determine if she is in remission. If she is in remission, the next phase of her treatment will commence.

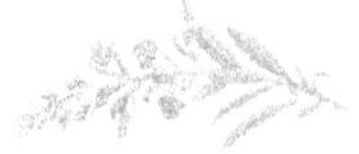

"

I think I first considered cutting my hair off about twenty minutes after that very first phone call from my pediatrician. *If Esther loses her hair, will she notice? Will it bother her? Will my hair being shaved or short help her? How good will I look with a pixie cut? Maybe this is the time for a daring hair decision.*

I'm sure you can all tell me I am not the first woman to consider a drastic haircut during a traumatic life event. Usually these sorts of haircuts are terrible choices and end with tears and uneven bangs. However, cancer is not your everyday traumatic event, and cutting one's hair in response to a loved one likely losing theirs involuntarily is not a bad idea.

Hair is a strange thing in the cancer world. I think anybody will readily admit, "It's just hair. It grows back." But this is not a helpful sentiment for a woman who has just made a terrible life decision, cutting her own hair for the first time via YouTube tutorial. It is likewise not helpful for somebody who has cancer. Or their mother, who cries as she finds sweet baby hairs literally everywhere but on the head of her child.

To shave or not to shave that tiny, perfect head? I suppose it depends. We chose not to. Have you ever tried shaving a rabid weasel? I didn't want to have a comparable experience to that. Losing hair wasn't bothering Esther, so if it bothered me, I could just deal with it like a grownup.

Well, it did bother me. Seeing the light glint off her head, which usually had about fifty frowsy strands clinging on in various places, was a hard and constant reminder of what we were facing. The port scar is usually covered by clothing. No matter how wide a headband is, that sweet, little, shiny head still pokes through.

Although, I will say, kissing that bald head was a strange silver lining. A friend told me I'd miss it. And while I don't know that I miss it yet, I didn't hate my lips touching that soft scalp skin.

(But maybe your teenager isn't so into you smooching their head, whether or not they have hair.)

I can't tell you what's right. But do what makes you and your kid the least stressed. Maybe now is the time to rock a bald head. It's definitely easier hair care. And it could be less distressing to shave it voluntarily instead of nursing those last few tender strands oh so carefully.

Esther was small enough that her bald head wasn't usually a point of comment. There are many children with unfortunate genes in the hair department. Usually the comments trended towards, "Oh, my child was as bald as an egg until they were three," or, "Don't worry, they all get hair eventually."

Sometimes I fumed; sometimes I let it roll off me. Usually I didn't say anything, because I try not to be a scene maker. The shocked and embarrassed look on people's faces is satisfying for a few moments, but then I feel compelled to further explain and reassure that she's doing as well as is possible.

I'm an empathetic apologizer. Sorry about that, I'm trying to work on it.

I did have one instance at a lake that sticks in my head as one of the times I gave into the temptation to explain. I was on the ground, wrestling my one-year-old out of a wet bathing suit and into dry clothing, trying to keep everything as decent and as hygienic as possible. A few middle-aged ladies walked by, and one of them jovially locked in on my bald baby and commented, "Looks like you got hit by the no-hair fairy!"

Hands full of slippery baby, I immediately replied in a calm, cool voice, "Actually, she got hit by the chemo fairy."

That quickness of reply can be a blessing and a curse. I've worked years to try to keep my wit in check, to make my responses without stabbing someone with the sharpness of my humor. The poor lady who had made the comment froze on her way to the parking lot, tripping over her words in an attempt to apologize as quickly as possible. I kept my dignity as I knelt on the ground and made those (relatively truthful) platitudes which would help restore her heartbeat to a more regular pace. "It's hard, but she's doing pretty well."

My friend Becky, who was with me along with her kids, told me I'd let the lady off too easily. A lot of parents with diagnosed kids would agree. We're a pretty protective bunch, easily steamed about injustices to our already cosmically wronged babies.

Sometimes people who know about the diagnosis, dear friends or relatives even, can get this fight-or-flight reaction going. I have heard numerous cures and natural remedies for cancer fighting. Every person in a cancer circle of influence has. All these miracle cures from well-meaning people whom I love. It's sometimes hard to process these sorts of perceived intrusions. *You don't think I want my child to be healed?*

Is my every spare moment not dedicated to thinking of and researching ways to lighten their load?

But I know they (mostly) stem from loving hearts and a desire to *do* something. I would want to do the same in that situation. If I stumbled across an article that included a plausible cancer fighter, I would want to pass it on. What if it were the one thing that made the difference?

Of course, on this side of the cancer fence, I know being the parent of a kid with cancer is overwhelming. There are a lot of choices. Mostly ones you cannot make without assistance from medical professionals. You have to choose to put your trust into the care team at the hospital, and that includes accepting that they know best. A lot of dietary options or other homeopathic remedies are fine to do in addition, but please always run things by your oncologist. I know doctors often seem focused on their particular specialty and appear to treat less holistically. I struggle with that sometimes. But at the end of the day, no matter how far into treatment your kid is, you are still essentially in triage mode. Getting rid of that cancer is the number one priority. Once treatment is complete (hopefully forever), other (sometimes also important) things can take precedence. But if you are convinced in your heart that essential oils and a dairy-free diet will help treat your child (and your oncologist has no objections), go for it. Just remember that a lot of new and "cutting edge" things that masquerade as natural remedies are not fully tested yet and may have negative effects as easily as positive ones.

I don't think there's a black and white guide to answering these sorts of comments and helpful asides. Go by the state of your heart. I don't mean to say, "Go where your heart leads you," because as we know, the heart is deceptive (Jer. 17:9) and kind of a bad thing to follow. I mean, were you answering honestly and conversationally to that comment about your kid's hair, or were you feeling angry and spiteful with a desire to wound? The same words and even the same tone can even come out from both heart states, but where you're coming from makes a huge difference.

You know where your heart is, and the Audience of One certainly does

***

One of the perceptions I've had to fight are my own. I read an article about casseroles,[1] and I have to admit that it's stuck with me. The general idea of it was, when hard times come, who gets a casserole from the Committee of Caring People at your church? Certainly us, in the early days of diagnosis. Probably us, if relapse or difficult side effects happen. The death of a spouse is grounds for a number of casseroles. Families with new babies definitely get several weeks of meals.

But what about a divorce, even a biblically condoned one? How about a family with a "severely" special needs child? What about the foster family that's spending months at a time in the pursuit of keeping their family from coming unglued? The way people see you and rate your supposed sufferings goes directly into their actions towards you. Which is why a little bald girl is given more pity and attention than a little girl with a full head of hair.

I would be remiss to write a book about our time in the Valley of Despair and not mention my friend, Becky. We moved to a little town called Xenia in Ohio a few months before Esther was born to accept Robert's position as pastor to children and their families at Dayton Avenue Baptist Church. Becky gave birth to her fourth child, Elaina, three weeks before Esther was born. We became good friends. Serendipity (and let's get real here, God) found us moving out of a rental and into a house directly next door to their family before Esther turned one.

1. Redtentliving.com/2019/09/13/the-casserole-rules

We found ourselves at each other's houses constantly. We borrowed cups and cups of sugar, enjoyed endless cups of tea together, and watched our kids begin the process of growing up together.

Their house and our house are pre-1900 era Victorian houses. Lots of character—both good and bad. Our houses are almost certainly built by the same builder, as they are almost perfectly mirror images of each other, inside and out. It seems like some sort of masterful literary device that so physical a thing should be indicative of our lives.

About the time that Esther was diagnosed, Becky's husband began working a second job to try to keep up with bills. His children did not see him, aside from a few hours on the weekend. Becky homeschools her kids, which means she went from having a few hours of respite in the evenings to almost constant, unrelenting mothering.

Four kids under age ten is a lot of responsibility on its own. When one of those kids is a mischievous toddler, and another is a preschooler who is lovingly referred to as a "Tasmanian Devil" by his mother, it can be overwhelming on a completely different level.

Becky did not get a casserole. She wasn't taking a kid to get chemo at the hospital, but she was juggling school, housework, special needs, a cake-baking business, and learning how to do everything via YouTube—from fixing car wiring to wielding power tools to mending broken appliances.

I compare our lives often. So different, and yet I'm sure that had we measured, our blood pressure surely would have been rising on the same days. When Esther was going through her initial tooth troubles, Becky had two kids with significant dental work done. Our bill got paid by Esther's insurance, because it is cancer related. Becky has significant copays from these incidents.

Life is just hard sometimes.

But we took the hint from God, who was so gracious to have given us houses literally so close that I can hear when Elaina is denied a second helping of dessert. We persist together, lean on one another, and bear burdens where we can. This is what community and family look like as Christians. We're not perfect, but we try to grow closer to God together.

I could tell you about more friends who struggled with their own things while we were going through Esther's cancer treatment. That would not be a challenge. I know I've said it, but I'll reiterate. A whole lot of people are going through hard times too. Pediatric cancer seems like the pinnacle of all tragedy, and in many ways, it is. But it should not elevate us to sainthood and certainly should not trivialize or overlook the sufferings of friends in our own backyard or across the world. Our world is full of sin and death. We don't have the monopoly on tales of woe.

Try to think about how others are feeling while they are thinking of you. Then work together. Pray for one another. It makes the world a nicer place.

> *James 5:13-16: Is anyone among you suffering? Let him pray. Is anyone cheerful? Let him sing praise. Is anyone among you sick? Let him call for the elders of the church, and let them pray over him, anointing him with oil in the name of the Lord. And the prayer of faith will save the one who is sick, and the Lord will raise him up. And if he has committed sins, he will be forgiven. Therefore, confess your sins to one another and pray for one another, that you may be healed. The prayer of a righteous person has great power as it is working.*

Dear Splitting Hairs,

I know there's a lot of controversy around being politically correct in your everyday actions. Is it OK to breastfeed in public? Is it okay to comment on said breastfeeding? If a man (who shall remain nameless) is growing his lovely, long, red hair long to donate, is it OK for little old ladies in the supermarket to tell him how beautiful it is?

He's weirded out by it, but I think that one is probably fine.

And is it OK for people to comment on your child's lack of hair? Or the accessed central line tube that is sticking out from the neckline of their shirt? Would you comment on an elderly gentleman using oxygen or a wheelchair?

Maybe. But probably not. I suppose I can think of a few very select instances where it might not be strange. ("Hey, I like your purple wheelchair! My grandma just has a black one, but she let me put a dinosaur sticker on it.")

Most people probably aren't trying to be offensive when they say things. We just all have this human condition where words come out of our mouths before we have time to consider them. Questions probably irk me less than an unsolicited comment; it's beautiful humanity that draws us to examine our fellow man instead of ignoring everyone until we can safely lock the door of our house behind us again. Our wonderful pastor likes to select the longest line at the grocery store, as to have the best chance of getting to know people and spreading the gospel of Jesus Christ.

I shamefully do not follow this excellent example. It's hard to get to know people as your toddler is having a screaming fit because the checkout line is too long.

But maybe instead of immediately leaning back on the comfortable, "I'm offended by what they just said," we can look for the opportunity of evangelism. How can we share the love of God and encourage?

I say all this as a reminder to myself as well as to you—because believe me, I am not holier than thou.

Love,

Hair Today, Gone Tomorrow

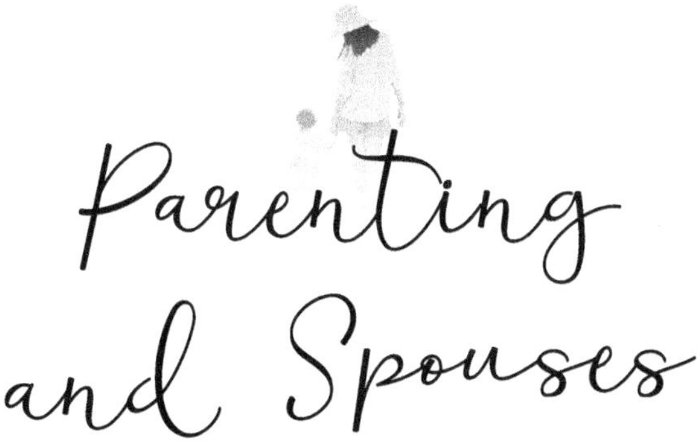

Parenting and Spouses

I dwell on the different experiences of big kids and little kids on the Hem/Onc floor. Both have cancer. Both likely have lasting physical and mental side effects, although they will likely present differently in every case. Moms of teenagers tell me they can't imagine the stress of chasing a fast little person with a needle stuck in their skin. I tell them I can't imagine the stress of having conversations about mortality with a teenager.

But there are similarities between your kid with cancer and my kid with cancer. They are uncertain; they are scared. They have pain and nausea. Questions and concerns bubble in their minds—they just come out differently. And how we deal with that energy is indicative of how we are raising our kids.

One of these technical terms I've come across is *emotional dysregulation*.[2] It fortuitously explains this very phenomenon that I have been mulling over here, proving that there are many, many smarter human beings than myself

2. Jessicalangtherapy.com/blog/regulate-relate-reason-brain-state/

in the world. But, as I'm the only one here (sorry about that), let me expound.

This dysregulation happens during times of sensory input, upsetting a child's balance. The past traumas that color the view your child has of the world bubble to the surface. Essentially, their alarm state has been triggered. During this, it's more of a challenge for them to behave appropriately, no matter the age. They will have trouble listening, comprehending, and dealing with the situation.

Parenting through this has been quite the interesting side quest. I won't pretend to be a parenting guru, as Esther is my first (and currently only) child. Parenting a toddler and parenting a teenager are two vastly different subjects, I'm sure. However, I think there is some small amount of overlap, so I'll share my imperfect pearls of wisdom.

Identifying your child's misbehavior (or actions in need of guidance) isn't always easy. However, one of the positives about spending so much time with them at the hospital is that you are almost one person now. Or close enough. A lot of the time, you can see where an outburst or a shutdown is coming from. You know when a reaction is normal and when it's exacerbated by the unfair lot that life has given them.

You, being a rational creature, possibly more intelligent than myself, know it's two different things entirely to parent or discipline in a moment of heightened, exaggerated emotion, or to do so when things are "normal." If it is a situation of the latter—well, sorry. I'm not going to help you parent in a normal way, because I am wildly underqualified. I have a bachelor's degree in digital media studies, not psychology or sociology. I feel like a charlatan trying to give you professional advice anyways, so I'm definitely not going to jump to your assistance in this one. Since I have endeavored to write a book on the subject of having a kid with cancer, I will take a stab at the other (i.e., parenting in exaggerated emotion).

One day, leaving the hospital after many hours of the usual fun, my child threw the biggest fit of her life. I was alone with Esther in the hospital lobby, surrounded by several dozen people. I couldn't hold her, because despite knowing she weighed 13.6 kg a few hours previously, she had increased in mass threefold since then.

I gripped her wrists tightly, and she hung from my hands like an enraged bull. Her feet were on the ground, yes, but she used those instruments to drum against the floor and occasionally pedal in the air. This is our tantrum position when out and about. I'm not going to let her press her face against any floor but our own. Yes, I am so, so mean.

At least six people I personally knew observed us while my little banshee made maximum benefit of the tall, acoustically resonant lobby ceiling. "Whose child is this?" I joked to each of them. All because I did not get her one of the helium balloons at the gift shop. Yes, they were shaped like animals. Yes, she said "pweeease?" in a manner that made my heart melt and want to immediately relent and spent twelve dollars on a scrap of mylar that would float around my house and end up scaring the poop out of me prematurely on a midnight bathroom excursion.

It was such a pristine example of a toddler moment. While others may have been in supreme embarrassment, I was in such a state of amusement that I fought to not let my child see the smile on my face. Because that would have disrupted the course of action I am about to propose to you.

Remember the three Rs: regulate, relate, reason.

Regulate. Soothe your child. Once Esther was calm enough to handle in my arms again, I held her close and stroked her hair with loving, motherly hands. I spoke in a soft voice that I would use if she were waking from a nightmare. You have to get them stable—this is triage. Make your child feel safe and loved.

Relate. You are with them all the time; you can reason out why they're acting the way that they are. Make them understand that you understand. "I know you really wanted that balloon. I know you've had a long, hard day. You've been such a big girl today. Mommy is so proud of you." (I understand an older kid may act like they resent being understood, but I think this is still a viable action. Modify it however you think will work for your child.)

And finally, *reason*. I find that relating and reasoning can sometimes happen together, depending on the circumstances. This is where you remind your child of the rules. "We don't throw fits. We use our words. We don't always get what we want." An older child is going to be swayed more by logic than my toddler. Little kids need you to continue using that calm, soothing voice, and repeat things in multiple ways that they've heard before and know to be statements of fact. You have to ground them where they're comfortable. If you're calm and certain, they will eventually mirror you.

Parenting is fun, huh? Desperately hoping you turn out a profitable member of society, as well as one with a good heart. Consistency is the bread and butter of successful parenting, and yet it's the one thing you can't be sure of in cancer treatment.

Cancer is (hopefully) temporary. You will have the rest of your kid's life to get them trained back to where you want them to be. Yes, you can have expectations of your cancer kid, but things are going to look different. I let Esther watch more TV when she's feeling bad. I give her greater latitude for her actions and "words." She's feeling like crap most of the time and handling it with a heck of a lot more grace than I would. Some things I address now, and other things I let slide. She needs the grace and understanding sides of love right now a little more than the discipline side.

That being said, I do think it's very important to have some boundaries. Yes, you need to love your child and give grace (both now and in regular non-cancer life). But the verb of *love* is not always pertaining to cuddles and extra helpings of ice cream.

Sometimes it's tough love. Not rushing your child's homework to school after them because they were careless and forgot it. Not letting your child get away with a knock-down drag-out temper tantrum because you're not going to McDonalds today.

Giving your child the latitude to become entitled and lazy is a slippery slope. It's one that we're all stumbling along, trying not to get pulled down too far. This is a difficult endeavor during the times you're trying to make up for painful port accesses and nauseating medications. But kids do crave boundaries (though it's few children who will understand or admit this).

You've probably been a parent longer than I have. But hopefully some of this resonates or helps.

> **May 25**
>
> ARA-C 3/4. Another relatively quick day—two hours. A sweet nurse, who we've had the last three days in a row, knew it was our anniversary, and had balloons and cupcakes and cookies waiting in our room for us. She went out of her way to get them for us herself, at a bakery near her house.
>
> The amount of love and care we receive at Dayton Children's is astonishing.
>
> Esther was feeling pretty low key yesterday, and she spent a fair amount of time sitting. She then had a low-grade fever most of the night, almost getting to the point of having to go in to the hospital. It hit 101 at one point, but after thirty minutes of waiting and praying, it went back down to normal. We are very thankful we got to stay in our bed at home.
>
> Chemo went well: Esther is feeling a bit tired but seems pretty happy as long as the mother ship is nearby.
>
> 

***

I call the hospital my personal spa, but still, it was a pretty unexpected way to spend our sixth wedding anniversary. When Robert and I repeated the timeless, "in sickness and in health," I don't think either of us had an inkling that it might relate to the oft devastating sickness of a child of ours, barely one year old. And while this book is about my child with cancer, I would be remiss to not spend at least a few sentences more talking about my husband.

In marriage, your relationship to your spouse should be placed above all others, except that with God. Even our delightful, tiny humans, who give us enormous joy and frustration, whom we pour vast amounts of money and mental sanity into, should not supersede the importance of your husband or wife. This is a hard lesson to follow, even without cancer and a sweet, sad child who begs to be indulged.

You can't "carve out time" like they always encourage you to do. Taking a regular date night seems laughable right now for any number or reasons. So, you get creative. That whole "intentional" part of marriage comes alive. After kid bedtime (the happiest time of the day!), you force yourself to cozy up to your spouse and have a conversation on the couch instead of staring blankly into space from across the room.

Well, maybe it's not such a burden. I do, after all, like my husband a bit.

And fortunately, I can boast (with only a little bias) of a loving and wonderful husband and that Robert still loves me and has patience with my manic mothering through these dark, confusing waters. As long as we have been in a relationship, my key word for him has been *safe*. I feel safe with him. I feel well cared for. I hope I can return this in whatever flawed way I'm able. Robert keeps our family steady and grounded. He checks his emotions and picks up the pieces of his hysterical daughter and wife on a regular basis. Even though lately, our newly verbal child has started to boss him around in a pretty humorous and rude way. I wonder aloud where she got it from, and he just looks at me with eyebrows raised.

When I ask him to do something, whether it be to take out the garbage or to take on the entire struggle of our insurance battle, he does it without question or sign of impatience. Well, maybe the occasional martyred sigh. But I'll let him have it.

Don't neglect your significant other. Kids aren't under your roof forever; you'll want something to talk about after they leave the nest besides, "Hey, remember all the times I ignored you because I was stressing about things I had no control over? Good times!"

Remember how kids need stability and grounding and consistency? Give them that gift, in your stable and strong relationship with your spouse (if you are so fortunate as to have one).

And if you are navigating all this as a single parent—bravo. I know you have no choice about it, but you're a superstar. I pray you have a strong village around you to lean upon. And perhaps read the next chapter about personal sanity, because I'm guessing it is more applicable to you than many.

Dear Master Juggler,

Welcome to the circus.

Take care of the relationships in your family. At the risk of sounding like a Wildcat, you're all in this together. Everybody is contributing in their own way, so recognize that. It's not easy on anybody. Keeping your communication open and honest is important. So many troubles of the Gilmore Girls would have been averted had there simply been more straightforward communication. I learn so much from Lorelei's mistakes.

Love,

Maybe One of Those Circus Animals Who Jumps Through Flaming Hoops for Treats?

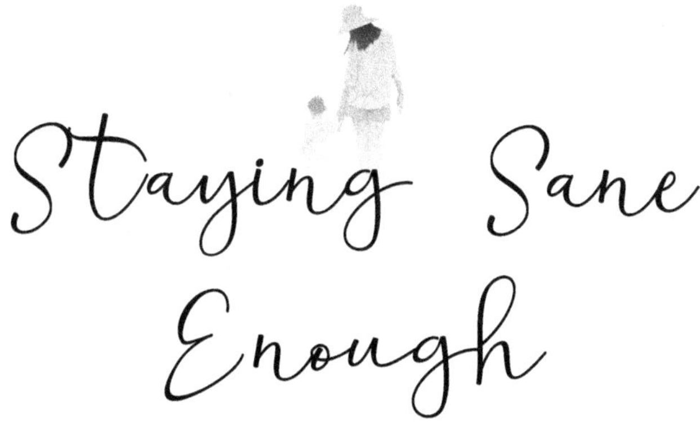

Staying Sane Enough

The first month was undoubtedly the hardest for me. And there was another memorable chunk of treatment where a short burst of steroids coincided with Erwinia; that was pretty terrible. But as time went on and we got closer to the maintenance phase of her treatment, I felt the strain acutely. I experienced a part of myself I had not yet encountered in twenty-eight years.

"Maintenance" was the final phase in Esther's B-cell ALL treatment. In her particular case, she had about ten months between her diagnosis and this phase. Instead of once a week treatment (or more), she would go down to once a month hospital visits for about two years.

I am a level-headed person. I, of course, have my share of issues, but I'm pretty mentally solid. But the last few months of frontline treatment before maintenance were *hard*. Why would nothing keep Esther from throwing up for twelve hours after Erwinia? How come she had this mysterious and frankly dreadful-looking rash on her legs?

May 3

Erwinia 6/6

Not our best day. Esther hasn't eaten anything and still started feeling bad pretty quickly. Did some throwing up. Currently having a doze on Grandma.

There's sometimes no rhyme or reason to the nausea. It's frustrating but there's nothing more we can do.

The dermatology saga continues as we try to get her in somewhere about her rash. I'm starting to learn that there are not enough dermatologists in the world.

Taking the steroids is still a struggle. And I lied in an earlier post: we're not done. They will make a reappearance in a few months.

After today, Esther gets her blood checked on Wednesday (5/8) and Monday (5/13). If all is well in those counts, we begin the second month of this phase on that following Wednesday (5/15). A whole lot of things will happen on that day: LP, various IV chemos, the beginning of a course of oral chemo. I won't overload you with that yet.

Finishing the steroid will not be restful, but after that we should have a bit of calm. Grandma and Grandpa will stay until next weekend, which will ease the difficulty of the steroid week somewhat.

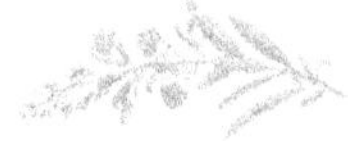

(Side note: apparently methotrexate can do that.) I was worn down after countless excursions to the hospital, months of terrible sleep, and enough stress to fill a decade. Yes, I'm clearly supermom (that's sarcasm), but even I have a breaking point.

It became hard to have fun at times and enjoy moments that were nice. I just wanted to curl up on the couch until it was all done.

But I'm a mom; I can't do that. You understand. There's laundry and food and, of course, the offspring factor. Not to mention those hospital visits that keep coming. You catch your breath after one treatment, your kid starts to feel like themselves for an hour or two, and that's when you cart them off for another dose of the poison that you hope is killing the cancer.

Life slips away from you slowly; odd jobs and chores pile up. And it's hard to face those things when you're busy dealing with more important things, so you just let them slide and live in a little bit of squalor for a season.

And that's OK. *Please give yourself grace, Mom.* I've said that before, but I want you to really hear it. I need to hear it myself. You can't do everything, but do what you can. Figure out what is doable, and do it. Make a list—conquer one thing at a time. My dad has a philosophy of doing at least three productive things in a day. Items can be as impressive as, "Cleaned behind the fridge," down to the mundane, "Brushed my teeth." Measure your success with a ruler befitting your circumstances.

Enlist some of your village to come help out. Maybe you have wonderful parents, like I do, who come to restore your sanity by cooking and cleaning for a week.

It's an amazing gift to have good people around, and I'll bet you do. But even if you don't, talk to the social worker at your hospital. They will be able to direct you to services and assistance that you are eligible for. A lot of people and companies want to help families in the midst of pediatric cancer. Don't be too proud if you need something. This is what those things are there for.

Be kind to yourself. Take an extra five minutes in the shower to enjoy the hot water. Have a can of soda instead of a healthier source of caffeine; it tastes good, and you need the energy, gosh darn it! Leave the kids at home with your husband or a friend, and go to the grocery store alone. It's a mom luxury, and you deserve it.

As humans, our sanity and general well-being are so precariously balanced—a fact that I remembered keenly during Esther's final few weeks of intense treatment. When two out of three nights' sleep are classifiable as "bad" due to my child feeling ill, the threat of vomit, or any number of other things, this in itself takes a toll on your physical and mental status. It's strange . . . I have to keep reminding myself that I am in a horrible situation, and it is OK to feel certain ways and act certain ways. It is OK to make allowances for myself and admit to others that it's been a rough morning. Some days, or stretches of days, are good. Even during treatment sometimes, in the face of puke, I am content and calm. The master of my emotions. But other times, during no discernible, unusually "bad" happenings, I struggle to make it. Planning supper and conversing casually seem like monumental feats, and I cannot fathom why. I beat myself up. And then I remember that my child has cancer, that I am making a full-time job out of her treatment while trying to be a wife and mother and do a part-time job of graphic design. I am also trying to have a life outside of the hospital, and this means I need to make meals and talk to people.

My life has become simpler in some ways. My priorities are honed. If I spend the day keeping my baby happy, as a mom of a newborn might spend months doing—then regardless of the size of the pile of unfolded clothes on the couch, I've done my job. It's a small weight off my burdened shoulders.

Giving myself permission to be "lazy"—aka recharge—is hugely freeing, and I recommend it highly. There is no day stormier (hopefully), so feel free to call in all your rainy-day cards. At times, I have eaten fast food two or three times a week for months, because "fies" (especially the Chick-fil-A variety) are one of the only things my kid eats reliably. And by golly, I'm going to fatten this kid up so she can take another beating with chemo and come out the other side functioning.

***

One of the places I found solace was in fellow "cancer moms" community. If you haven't heard of Momcology,[3] stop reading right now and go find it. It's a support group run by fellow mother warriors, functioning on many levels. Local chapters meet for coffee and laughs over port malfunctions. Online groups are there to fill in the gaps—and there are so many gaps, once you start looking. I didn't know I needed a place where someone could share a photograph of a weird face rash on their kid and have ten people within an hour assuring them it's probably a methotrexate rash. But here we are.

I didn't find my way to the Facebook groups until well over a year past Esther's diagnosis. Immediately I saw the benefit and had a sudden need to reach out and look for somebody, anybody, who was in a similar boat with breastfeeding. This was initially hard, as I'm definitely a lurker on public pages.

But I was at the end of my rope. No one I knew at the hospital was still breastfeeding. Most of my friends with non-sick children weren't doing much breastfeeding past the age of two. Even those wonderful "crunchy" friends were beginning to see their little ones taper off naturally. Esther continued to frantically want to nurse a dozen times a day and more often in the night. I slept, most nights, curled around her as she snuggled into me. Sweet, but being awakened six to eight times in a normal night takes a toll on your sanity. I began to doubt the damage it was doing to my mind and body and wondered if this was normal "mom tired." Either way, I couldn't conceive of a world where I tried to even partially wean her anytime soon. She needed me.

3. Momcology: momcology.org.

I needed to find somebody who understood. Continuing was the impossible I had to do, because the alternative was even more unthinkable. But I needed somebody, just one person, to stand up and say, "I get it. I've been there."

So I found courage, and I posted to the main Momcology group.

The response was immediate and overwhelming. Within an hour, twenty people had responded to me. Within a day, over fifty people had taken time out of their lives to spend paragraphs in descriptions of their like circumstances, commiseration, and encouragement.

"

Feb 9

I suppose I'm looking for a little solidarity today from fellow moms breastfeeding their CK (cancer kid). Esther is almost 2.5 (was diagnosed with ALL just after her first birthday, and we've still got 1.5 years of treatment) and is pretty obsessed with mama milk.

We co-sleep, and many nights I'm positive she is attached to me all night. During the day, she's nursing quite a bit. It's a lot on me physically (I think I'm always exhausted and don't realize it) and mentally (she's pretty attached to me and mostly me—makes having solitary introvert time tough).

It feels like such a small inconvenience compared with everything else, and I don't like to make a big deal about it. But I feel so far removed from everyone I know in person, even my crunchy mom friends who BF a long time. I just can't compare it to anything.

I'm not looking to wean (the nutrition, immunity, and comfort are too good to not!), but I think I just need some virtual hugs from other moms in the same boat. I think this might be the right place to find my peeps.

"

I cried. I read comment after comment of women who I have never met in my life, pouring out this quiet, private part of their lives to me.

I'm not alone. I'm not alone.

I drank in these life stories, so many of them starting with, "I could have written this." To know that I was blessedly one of many filled a gap that I didn't realize was there. I didn't know that the solidarity would feel like a physical buoyancy of my soul, attaching a helium balloon to my core emotions for every woman that said, "I've been there too."

It might not be breastfeeding a toddler with leukemia. Maybe it's an eight-year-old with a tumor and autism. Maybe it's the sibling of your CK, struggling in school on top of everything. Or maybe it's something your humble author cannot even conceive of.

It doesn't matter. Because beautifully and unfortunately, you are not alone in that impossible thing that is your Everest. Almost certainly, someone has done it before or is going through it now. Even if your struggle is pinpoint specific to you and your family, I guarantee that the base elements of it will be relatable to someone.

Please do not be like me and wait too long to find community or therapy. Nobody is so good or sane that it is dismissible.

Dear Mom Bun,

I love your hair. I relate to that messy "do" on a deep level, even though I chopped off two feet of hair in the hospital and only have enough left to make stubby pigtails. I also love your sweatpants—and tight sweatpants that we call "leggings" or "yoga pants" . . . like the name makes the unidentifiable stains and food handprints less visible. They are ridiculously comfortable, and you look your best when you're comfy.

You are looking great, by the way. I'm sure you've showered within the past month and have definitely had a cup or two of caffeine today, so you're also functioning.

I love that you haven't cleaned your bathroom in a while. The toothpaste splatter on the mirror obscures your face just enough that you can blame any shortcomings of your appearance on good dental hygiene. What a model of humanity and beauty you are!

Your kids look pretty happy. You are a great mom, letting them eat junk and watch a movie in the middle of the day. I challenge you to be an even better mom, and make it a double feature next time. Feel free to encourage all-day pajamas as a part of the party.

No words of advice in this little note. I've bossed you around enough in the rest of this thing. Just wanted to let you know that you are beautiful, and you are a great mom.

Love,

Messy Hair Don't Care

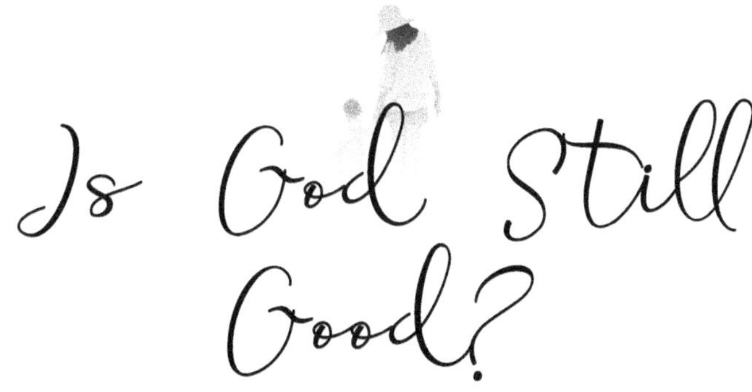

Is God Still Good?

The way I look at God and the world has changed. The angle from which I view things has altered slightly but suddenly and leaves me asking questions over again—ones that I thought had resolved.

Is God good?

Well, let me get right to it here. Yes. The answer is yes. This was a question I asked early in Esther's diagnosis and one that I answered like breathing. *Yes, God is good.* Maybe I understand that goodness a little differently now. It's a little deeper. God's goodness is not dependent on me or my circumstances but on Him and His ever-abiding character. I see the way He preserves us and carries us, when all earthly strength is gone.

> *1 Chronicles 16:34: "Oh give thanks to the Lord, for he is good; for his steadfast love endures forever!"*

Psalm 145:8-9: "The Lord is gracious and merciful, slow to anger and abounding in steadfast love. The Lord is good to all, and his mercy is over all that he has made."

It would be easy to see the situation through a lens where my little one was robbed of her babyhood. Where I wonder about an "alternate dimension Esther" who never had those cancer cells mutating in her body. What sort of life does that little girl lead? What are the things my Esther is missing out on?

Probably not much. She lives a pretty full life. Fuller and richer sometimes, even because of her hospital escapades. If you can believe it.

"

May 24

We left at 8:45 last night, got home at 9:15, and Esther threw up spectacularly all over our front porch.

We're trying a new approach to discouraging solicitors. Spaghetti strawberry chemo puke. Sorry. I know that is way more than you wanted to know!

But we dosed her with Zofran, gave her the oral chemo, and she went right to bed. All slept well.

We woke up and came back to the hospital for an 8:30 appt. At 9:50, her ARA-C got started, and it is just a fifteen minute one. We should be out of here momentarily. Then back tomorrow morning for another short appt.

"

It would also be easy to be bitter towards other people. To see the small sweetnesses and accomplishments of other little ones and watch their untainted lives with jealousy. To put an ominous shadow on their sunshine, foretelling doom and destruction for their future. Because nobody is allowed to remain happy. Something will happen to twist this innocence into a tragedy.

This is, of course, absurd. Not everyone experiences an event like this. And even if something hard happens, it is never exactly like anyone else's. Bad things don't happen because someone was especially bad or good or even because there was an excess or void of difficulty already present. One of our friends at the hospital is a hypoglycemic diabetic teenager with leukemia. Her house was destroyed by a tornado a few months into her treatment. It is not her fault. Trying circumstances are a result of the fallen nature of humanity. We are defiant and deserving of death in the face of a perfect God who cannot tolerate sin.

> *Romans 6:23: "For the wages of sin is death, but the free gift of God is eternal life in Christ Jesus our Lord."*

But God cares for us. He provides a reckoning for our sin. He gives grace even beyond that immeasurable love of paying the ultimate price for our own sin.

And we cannot judge the lives of others based on what we see. It's not logical. Other people have their own difficulties; whether or not they're harder than ours is not mine to know or say. And other people surely looked at us and compared their sorrows to our happiness. Maybe even still.

We all have a time for joy and a time for difficulty. We don't get to pick what "bad things" happen to us. We only get to choose how we react to them. (Didn't Gandalf say something like that?) It is not my job to resent people with supposed normalcy. I don't know their hearts. Aslan would tell me that it's not my story. It's not fair to judge based on what I see. And it's not up to me to give out good and bad lots in life, thank goodness. Sometimes I start to play the "what if" game and try to think what I'd do to not have this happening to my sweet baby. To me. What price would I be willing to pay? I quickly see the depth of my selfishness and am again thankful to God for not giving me that power.

Living at peace with this situation doesn't mean that we cancer moms aren't different. We are different because the world thinks of our suffering as being generally greater than its own. It is such a big *different* that people can't help but stop and stare and feel pity. It's like seeing a one-legged man or a homeless person. Most people feel pity but also thankfulness for their own two legs and sturdy house. And many seek out a way to help. Those people are set apart because they are viewed differently.

Standing on this side of the pity fence, I can tell you that yes, having a child with cancer is hard. But it doesn't make me a saint or an "amazing mom," as many people tend to put it. I'm just doing the best I can with the situation I'm in. I think that's essentially what good mothers everywhere do. But to my dear friends who call me an amazing mom—thank you for your hearts of encouragement. It does help me to hear those words of affirmation, a confirmation that my hard season is not going unnoticed.

Missionaries are another group of people who are viewed differently. Super Christians who live in a different country—what's less relatable than that? As a child of missionaries, I find many strange similarities between these two odd circumstances of my life. I want to discuss pieces of my life, past and present, but my terminology is out of sync with the rest of my peers.

Them: "This one time in Virginia . . ."
Me: "This one time in Hong Kong . . ."

> Them: "My toddler is getting so sassy!"
> Me: "Mine too! She said the funniest thing to a nurse at the hospital the other day."

Not everyone has an outlier situation, like living overseas or having a child with chronic illness. So it can be hard to relate to others without bringing the conversation to a screeching halt.

If you haven't already tried it, laughing over hospital shenanigans tends to make people laugh nervously and say, "aww," and conversation stumbles to an end. My only advice is to keep on plugging away at it. Find some good friends who understand you're not looking for pity or accolades. You're just looking to talk about what's going on in your life right now, like every other person on this planet. I would almost say it's more important for you to talk about your life to others; it keeps you less isolated and is a good outlet.

Regardless of how many people I talk to, I find myself talking to God more. I'll say this for pediatric cancer: it has exploded my prayer life. Not just for my child but for a whole plethora of little friends we've met through this journey—not to mention other people in hard circumstances that I suddenly resonate with.

Before I go to bed at night, I find myself reciting the names of little ones we've met at the hospital, thinking of their little faces. And I pray for specific children having more acutely difficult times.

> *Dear God, please let each of them live long and healthy lives on this earth. Let the cancer go away and never come back. Please let their long and healthy lives be spent loving You and glorifying You and serving You. Please let Your name be known through each of these stories; let Your glory be the epicenter. Let each of these kids' friends and family know that You are the reason for goodness. Please let their living lives be more glorifying to You than an early end.*

I pray this for my own daughter, and I feel that since the hospital is my mission field, it's my duty and privilege to cover every kid I can think of in prayer. I can't pray for every suffering kid in the world, and it wrecks me. But I can pray for these kids. Especially my own. God entrusted me with Esther. It is my job to take care of her physically, mentally, spiritually.

Knowing the words to pray is sometimes hard—a reality that would have surprised me before this all began. You're talking to God, what could be easier? Thank Him for goodness. Repent of sin. Ask humbly for what you desire.

That last one gets complicated. I desire my child to live. But doesn't every mother? Doesn't every mother pray this prayer? But not every child lives. And you can't pin it to a parent not praying, because sometimes the boldest prayer warriors are the ones whose prayers are not answered how they desired. So, what then? What's the key? What specific formula can I follow to ensure that my child survives this?

Sometimes I pray carefully crafted prayers, wording them to hem God in. *In order to answer this prayer, He* must *do it how I desire.* But God is not a computer, awaiting precisely worded code in order to spit out the correct programming. *He is God.*

When I pray, I sometimes pray for God's will. And then immediately after, I pray,

But if it's possible to let it turn out how I want also . . .

Oh, how often I do that. But how did Jesus pray?

Luke 22:42: "Not My will, but Yours."

The "but" that Jesus prays is really how I should be praying.

There are no magic words—no mystic rain dance that will force God to keep my little one alive. I can ask for things, and I *should* ask for things (1 John 5:14; James 5:16; Hebrews 4:16). God desires that we make our requests known to Him. And He does listen! He does consider our requests. I look at the story of Abraham, looking for a righteous man in Sodom and Gomorrah (Genesis 18:22-33). I look at Moses pleading for God to change His mind and have mercy on the Israelites (Exodus 32:11-14). Father God *loves* us deeply, intensely, passionately. He wants to give grace and show mercy. Parenting a child is a beautiful metaphor of this relationship.

> *Matthew 7:11: "If you then, who are evil, know how to give good gifts to your children, how much more will your Father who is in heaven give good things to those who ask him!"*

Are more fervent prayers more powerful? Is having such strong emotions creating a better, more heard prayer? I imagine the worst multiple times a day and pray with tears streaming down my face, begging the Lord to be merciful to me. *Please, Father. Indulge this mother. Be gracious, more gracious than you've already been. Give me what I don't deserve, again. Please.*

I dwell on this fervency of prayer question. Do I need to think about the worst-case scenario, let the emotions and fear overwhelm me, so I can pray with the most authentic and fervent emotions? We're told to not be fearful or anxious. To do so would be a distrust of God's sovereignty and ability. So where's the line? Clearly to be trustful of God. But I can't imagine praying emotionless.

> *Philippians 4:6-7: "Do not be anxious about anything, but in everything by prayer and supplication with thanksgiving let your requests be made known to God. And the peace of God, which surpasses all understanding, will guard your hearts and your minds in Christ Jesus."*

It comes down to one thing: I don't want to pray out of a sense of fear. I want to pray out of faith.

Is faith head or heart? I think it is neither; it is soul. And that is why it is such a hard thing to pin down. Trust comes from the head and heart working together, but faith is a deeper substance. It is the belief that God can and will work. Even if it is not always in the way you expect. But the place you feel it is your soul, which is maybe a combination of head, heart, and something else; the deeper substance that is you. That part of God breathed into you.

Faith is not the head knowledge that the percentages are in your favor, nor is it an emotional response—not entirely at least. How do I know I'm having faith? Those fleeting moments when I really *feel* it, deep in my being. As soon as I try to analyze where it's originating, it's gone, and I'm left wondering where my faith is and if I'm trusting for the right reasons.

> *Hebrews 11:1: "Now faith is the assurance of things hoped for, the conviction of things not seen."*

Life is a journey. There's not a pinnacle. You're always climbing, always learning.

***

As I have walked you through these pages and chapters, I speak of your kid's cancer like they're going to recover. I hope and pray that this is the case, just as you do. I don't think speaking positively about recovery or remission is a bad thing, until you know the time has come for other conversations, provided your child is mature enough to understand on some level.

I pray that each of you reading this book would already know that Jesus is our good Savior who died on the cross for our sins. And He rose again! And all we need do to ensure eternal life with Him is "confess with your mouth that Jesus is Lord" and "believe in your heart that God raised Him from the dead" and "YOU WILL BE SAVED!" (Romans 10:9). What an amazing Father He is.

Speak about these things with your child: the constant and eternal nature of God, not the frightening, shifting sand of humanity and life on earth. Whether or not things are dire, God is good. He expects and deserves our love and obedience through good times and bad; His goodness can be manifested in times of plenty or famine. Don't confine Him to being a deity of only sunshine-filled days or ignore Him unless you are in great need. Inconsistency does not become us! God deserves better. The best.

Friend,

No irreverent banter at the end of this chapter. Wholeheartedly, seriously, I hope you are already a believer in Christ or considering the matter with the gravity that it deserves. This book was born out of a horrible circumstance, but I hope that you see that my heart in this is not to punch you in the face with a Bible because I'm uneducated or blind to "real life" outside of faith and church matters. I live in the world, but I am not of the world. I am a child of the One True God, of the Great I Am. I am blown away by the magnitude of this privilege.

The Bible is truth. But my book isn't a book to try to convince you of that necessarily, though I think there are many other people, better theologically trained, who have authored books to this purpose. No, my reasoning is straightforward, and I will be honest with you. (1) I want to encourage you in this cancer parent business and remind you that you are not alone. (2) I want to educate you in a small way on some basic parts of this journey. (3) I want you to see that I have survived a while in this nightmare and still hold fast to the promise of God.

Abigail

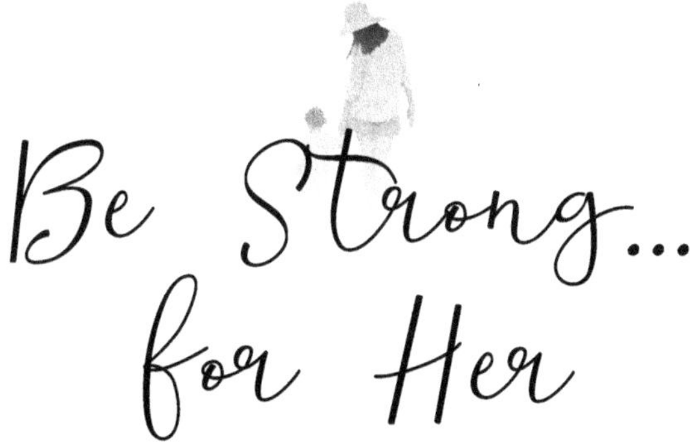

Be Strong... for Her

One of the first days we were at the hospital, I had a breakdown. Yes, I'd cried about once an hour since I got that horrible (yet fortuitous) phone call, but this was different. I stood in my child's hospital room, where three different nurses pinned down my one year old on that cage-like crib mattress. Her new port was giving them trouble, and they had to change out her needle.

"You can leave if you want," the nurses told me.

"No," I retorted. But my heart was shaky within me. We had already been through this, and I knew it was going to be drawn out and awful. Ten seconds in, I was brimming with tears, unable to take it anymore. But I had to be strong! I couldn't leave!

Robert could see beyond my "soldier mom" expression and told me to go. "It's fine," he said, holding her little hand. "I'll be with her."

He was a pillar of tearless strength, clasping our terrified child's hand with every ounce of fatherly love that he could muster.

And I fled from the room like a heartless chicken, hating myself entirely. I hated that I was not strong enough to stay, knowing she was not allowed to leave. I hated that the process wasn't giving us a break, complications arising where they needn't. I hated the cancer.

But mostly, in that moment, I hated myself.

I stumbled down the hallway, eyes downcast, hoping not to meet anyone's gaze or catch anyone's attention. I couldn't really see anyway—just enough to get past the nurses' station and duck into an empty conference room where I sought a chair at the far end of the room and dropped into it with the full weight of my body. Immediately I curled my legs up onto the chair, tucking my knees under my chin. I hugged my legs close, head down, leaning sideways onto the back of the chair. I had to make myself small. Crunch the misery up as little as it would get. If I squeezed myself enough, I wouldn't feel anymore. I just had to minimize my body and never release it again. Push my body in on itself, so eventually my broken heart could be forced back together.

But my mind roamed free. I called myself a coward, hearing the screams of my child in my ears even though she was too far away to hear. *What right do I have to run away when she was required to endure it? What kind of a pitiful excuse for a mother am I? And why is this happening to us?*

Why do bad things happen? I know the book of Job—seeing him live a cursed existence while God seemed to stand by and watch impassively. But God answered Job in the end, speaking out of the whirlwind.

> *Job 38:4: "Where were you when I laid the foundations of the earth?"*

Who am I, a product of God's grace and goodness, to question His actions and seeming inaction? He is greater than I.

> *Job 40:2: "Shall a faultfinder contend with the Almighty? He who argues with God, let him answer it."*

I am a vapor. A small, ephemeral piece of this temporary world. It is not my job to question but to obey—and honor God while I do so.

Sometimes it doesn't seem like a very satisfying answer. Thirty-eight chapters of watching Job suffer, and you'd think that there would be a pithy one-verse sum-up that we could put on T-shirts. Something that we can easily tell our friends: "See? Here's the answer. God has a plan."

But we read the Bible and see that God *does* have a plan. We sinned at the beginning, using our free will wrongly. And so the world is flawed. Earthquakes destroy cities, countries go to needless war, and innocent babies get cancer.

BUT GOD.

> *Ephesians 2:4-10: "But God, being rich in mercy, because of the great love with which he loved us, even when we were dead in our trespasses, made us alive together with Christ—by grace you have been saved—and raised us up with him and seated us with him in the heavenly places in Christ Jesus, so that in the coming ages he might show the immeasurable riches of his grace in kindness toward us in Christ Jesus. For by grace you have been saved through faith. And this is not your own doing; it is the gift of God, not a result of works, so that no one may boast. For we are his workmanship, created in Christ Jesus for good works, which God prepared beforehand, that we should walk in them."*

I cried alone for a time. My logical brain can't help me out with that. Sometimes you just have to cry.

Soon, my mom came in. She quietly walked over toward her baby, wrapped her arms around me and held me tightly—as if she was trying to shoulder some of my pain. A mother's embrace is a mysterious force; it has the power to heal a scraped knee, mend a broken heart, or dry up a tear-stained cheek. As this force began to work through my own tears, I managed to unravel my body from the cocoon I had forced myself in, pick myself up off the chair, and walk back toward my daughter's room. When I got there, I never walked out of her room again. My baby deserved a mom who was as strong as the one I have.

Sometimes you cry and break down and aren't the mom you want to be for your child. I suppose that's true in every circumstance of mothering, not just cancer. But when things are much worse, your failings seem much worse too.

I don't have a clear-cut answer, and I wouldn't dare suggest a perfect course of action. I would encourage you to stay strong, but give yourself grace. Cry if you need to, but know that your child draws strength from you. Be the stability they need by staying positive. But be the vulnerability they need by keeping your heart open.

Be a comfort to your child, not a stressor. Be a comfort to yourself also.

Use your mom instincts. Speak up when you have that feeling.

Pray often.

Aim to not only *survive* but to *thrive* through this affliction with which you've been appointed.

Strong One,

More than at any other point in your parenting career, doing what is best for your child is so extremely important. But I know you know that. I could urge you to stay in the room for hard things; I might discuss the merits of giving 110 percent and being present always, instead of checking your phone every so often.

But I know that life is not straightforward, and having one more person telling you what you're doing wrong as a parent is not helpful. Even I have been known to check my phone once or twice . . .

I will say, though, that though I see some parents declining to be in the room for accessing or other hard moments, I later see them evolving in their own journeys. As time goes on, they eventually start to stay. Whether or not this is how your progress as a parent looks, I'm not to say. But I can promise that you will grow, not shrink. Because you were made to be the caretaker of this child. And I know you're strong.

Love,

A Recovering Phone Addict

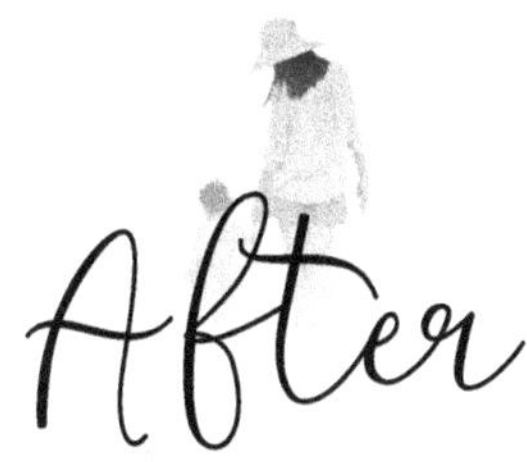

After

A lot of people, including you at first, will not understand how hard the "easy" part of treatment can be. Or the immediate aftermath of treatment—whatever the "step down" portion of the protocol is. Some things will be simpler and less overwhelming, but other things will rush in to fill the void. It might be that you can suddenly focus on your other children who desperately need much time and attention. Or your affected child may be needing extended PT or OT for the effects of chemo no longer in use. Possibly, the reality of what you've just survived will come crashing down around you, leaving you with unfathomable feelings and thoughts to wrestle through.

"

Nov 7

This little friend is doing so well. The first two weeks of every month are (we are discovering) going to be a little difficult, thanks to chemo IV/LP side effects, and then the steroids and aftermath.

Those steroids are hard.

But even through the steroid-enhanced toddler tantrums, Esther continues to grow and thrive. She's right in the middle of her month right now. We went to PT today, and her therapist is thrilled with Esther's energy level and progress. So much so that we're skipping the next appointment and coming back in a month to reevaluate her schedule.

Next week on Thursday we were fortunate to get an appointment with a pediatric dentist to assess Esther's teeth. She's got some enamel erosion on the front teeth, which, of course, is not what you want. Cause unknown, but likely a combo of many things. We're pretty good at wrestling her down and brushing, so it's not a lack of hygiene!

Please pray:

1. For no anxiety for Esther. She's not thrilled with the hospital these days. I don't know what she will do with an unfamiliar environment of the same ilk. Maybe I should find a Daniel Tiger episode or something . . .
2. For an easy solution and easy treatment scheduling. I assume she'll need to be put under for the fix, and if we can line it up with an existing LP, that'll be best.
3. For no insurance struggles. As long as "cancer" gets slapped on the diagnosis in the paperwork, BCMH should cover 100%.
4. For no current pain or long-term issues.

Thank you, friends! I'll keep ya updated.

”

I'm just tired. So tired. I wish I had some free time. It seems like a stupid and petty thing to desire when my child is responding to treatment so well, and treatment is lessened. But my tiny person, resilient but human, is battling whatever psychological damage she is constantly building by needing me close. Even Daddy or Grandma or Grandpa will not do for long; Mama must be there. Precious hours in the evening, between her bedtime and mine, are not exempt. She stirs and cries as she realizes the source of comfort is not at hand, and my time to work is punctuated by trips back and forth from my desktop to the bedroom—to nurse her, to stroke the inch of fine growth on her head, to curl my body protectively around hers.

Sometimes, for the third or fourth trip back of the night, I slam my mouse down in frustration. *I just need to work. I have so much to do.* I don't even get to my pile of "fun" things I'd like to do. I can't even scrape the bottom of my work pile. I can't catch my breath; I can't keep up. Leisurely things I used to do to cultivate superficial happiness gather dust; months and months stretch between the times I help Mario rescue Princess Peach. And my work is fragmented and not the quality I'd love it to be. Because my toddler can't give me a few hours—or even ten minutes—at night some nights.

Here's the reality: my baby doesn't get time off from cancer. It's in her body (or, it was), and she can't separate life with and life without because all her memories and moments come with that caveat of leukemia. There's no escape.

She's a baby. As I stand outside our bedroom, preparing to go in, I take a deep breath and change my attitude. I have to transform from selfish human to caring mother. My sweet, sweet small Esther does not understand the complexities of life—that I'm trying to keep working, because quitting a job that I enjoy would be financially foolish. She doesn't know that Mommy would desperately like to draw or paint for fun, because introverts need that time for mental stability.

All Esther knows is that in the dark of night, she wakes and reaches her arm out and can't find her mom, no matter how much she flails and flops. Her mom is a pillar of stability and comfort in this stormy sea of life, even more than a regular toddler would feel. I'm there when they start chemo, do blood pressure, give her stuffed animals. I'm holding her the moment she is put under sedation for a lumbar puncture and am at her side as soon as she begins to stir after.

Your story and your kid are different. But if I could guess, you've strengthened your bond and are a new kind of parent now. Your little one's trauma and methods of "dealing" might look different, but you're a rock in their storm.

It's hard to be that strong when you feel about as tough as cooked spaghetti. And it's hard to accept that after so many months or years, the factory settings on your life have not been restored.

***

As a sidebar, I want to say that I have gained a lot of respect for parents with medically challenging kids—parents who don't have the luxury of dog-paddling wildly to keep afloat until they reach the end of treatment. Some kids require 24/7 treatment for their whole lives. I have the (potentially misleading but still encouraging) light at the end of the tunnel. I can mark a date on a calendar and say, "If all goes according to plan, this is the last day my child gets primary treatment."

Cystic fibrosis. Untreatable tumors. Some physical ailments have no proven cure. Severe mental illness. Abuse victims. Parents of children with these ailments have a lot of sweet and triumphant moments that outsiders can't begin to understand. But they undeniably have a burden of stress that is equally incomprehensible.

I won't go on. I am not qualified to talk about this and will only put my foot in my mouth if I try to expound. So please take this message from my heart with the honor and respect I mean to convey. I know for many, every day is physically and mentally demanding for the kid and their parents. Hats off to you guys. You certainly deserve a shout out.

***

The aftermath of a natural disaster is akin to what you're experiencing. The flood waters have receded, aid has been distributed, and people know you've had a hard time. You have a temporary roof over your head, and friends have given you food and clothes. But enough time has passed that you and some other people may be thinking it's time for normal responsibilities to resume. You have to go back to work—begin operating your life as you had been previously. Yet you're still looking for a new permanent home, you're trying to scrape together enough time and money to replace clothes and furniture. And in the midst of it, your heart is in your throat every time it rains.

People are still there for you in a moment when you ask for help or prayers. But it's not going to be second nature anymore. People assume after a year or two that you're pretty self-sufficient. More dangerously . . . *you're* going to assume you can go back to normal life as it was. But the reality is, you're going to be dealing with the fallout from this your whole life.

When you lose an arm, you have to reevaluate the way you physically (and emotionally) interact with the world. In the same way, as soon as that cancer test comes back positive, your lens with which you view the world will be scarred and the way you approach the world will be different, likely for the rest of your life.

***

My husband is a children's pastor, and together we teach a class of first through third graders during one of the Sunday school hours. Well, he teaches, and I do "hanging out" and general crowd control. OK, mostly I create more distraction. Robert goes through the books of the Old Testament, and I ask if anybody has siblings named Habakkuk or Haggai.

One Sunday recently, he was sharing with the kids the story of the man blind from birth. (A lot of times, when we hear a story we've heard, it's easy to tune it out. Truthfully, I'm often in policing mode during class and am not always engaged in the story. *But it doesn't matter, right? This is a kids class. I can't possibly get anything out of it.*) In John 9, we see the account of Jesus healing this man who was blind from birth. His disciples asked who sinned, the man or his parents, to be born in such a way.

> *John 9:3: "Jesus answered, 'It was not that this man sinned, or his parents, but that the works of God might be displayed in him.'"*

I don't blame myself for Esther getting sick—at least, not usually. Her whole upbringing (starting from the womb) was pretty close to ideal, sometimes unnecessarily so. I craved noodles in a fierce way while pregnant, and I wouldn't let myself have more than a taste of instant ramen. So many preservatives and chemicals! I cried, but I didn't eat them. And when she was born, she was breastfed. When she started to eat, I gave her good fruits and vegetables. Healthy grains. Nothing loaded with sugar. Our house was smoke-free. My cleaning chemicals were limited. She didn't crawl away and lick the bathroom floor. I only had one kid to watch, and by golly I was going to do it well.

And yet, she got cancer at an impossibly young age. Did I do something else wrong? A sin that caused God to shake His head regretfully and smite my child with this disease? No, and neither did *she* do anything. It just happens.

Hear me, friend. I don't know if you struggle with feelings of guilt. But if you do, please stop. Cancer can come for anyone. A lot of the time, as with many other illnesses and disorders, we cannot know what brought it about. You're doing a good job caring for your little person (and any others you have). Don't waste time and energy on guilt.

> *". . . but that the works of God might be displayed in him."*

What a blow of encouragement. In that classroom, as I whispered for kids to face forward and sit on their bottoms, I was hit with this unexpected revelation of purpose. We have been given this opportunity that we may proclaim the glory of God. I've been trying to look at this suffering through a lens of thankfulness, but to see it spelled out and exampled so clearly in scripture was an encouragement I did not expect to get that day.

Of course, it's easy to feel self-righteous on a day like today, when my child is happy and in a much less rigorous section of treatment. It's a different story when my child is throwing up and her future seems uncertain. I'm fighting every moment then to not be panicky and whiny in the valley. And those are the glamorous times! People remember to pray better during the days of really difficult treatment. Your suffering is on a pedestal. It's new. It's fresh. Prayers and physical help tend to run the most enthusiastic with these heightened emotions novelty brings.

When a year passes, and the treatment is still hard, it's a different story. It's easy to be forgotten or dismissed. After all, the chemo is less frequent, less harsh. Esther's hair is growing back in, finally. The little port scar on her chest—which, for whatever reason, brings me to this visceral reaction of sadness—has faded. I want to compulsively trace the tender, now-healed line of scar, running my fingers along its length and mourning the marring of perfection. To feel the hard intrusion of necessity just under her skin, through which endless hours of chemo have coursed. But I don't. I stare at it; I imagine how it would feel beneath my fingertips. I know touching it will trigger emotions in my child, emotions she can't quite grasp the enormity of, but ones she can most certainly feel. She can comprehend fear.

The fear isn't gone, but it has faded. We are moving on and forward. Other people are too.

I'm convicted about how often I've slowly stopped praying for or "checking up" on someone after a miscarriage, a divorce, or a parent has passed away. I've been fortunate enough not to have experienced these things, and it's easy to assume things are better because you don't see them crying in the hallways at work. But I know, when I take the time to really ponder these things, that they don't magically get better. Those are the scars you carry with you; everybody has them to some degree. They just look different on everyone.

Most people don't have the luxury of a social media page devoted solely to their suffering. I know if I make it known that we're struggling for whatever reason, there are several hundred people ready to drop to their knees before the throne of God on our behalf. *If I'm brave enough to post it.* And if I don't, there are still countless lovely people—some of whom I have not met—who pray for us faithfully daily.

There's another example for you of truly being blessed.

You've noticed a common theme of "other people" in our story. Even though it's "just" Esther and me at the hospital—it's really not. There is a team of medical professionals there. A whole second family of beautiful kids and parents who also live their second lives on the Hem/Onc floor. And when we come home, my wonderful, irreplaceable rock of a husband is there to stabilize my emotions, make us feel loved, and clean up puke. My parents drive six hours to us at least once a month to take away all my household responsibilities—except for mothering my child. My sister sends gifts and love and fudges the numbers on our joint cell phone bill so we don't have to pay as much. Friends from afar send money and gifts and an endless line of Chick-fil-A gift cards. Friends nearby are there in a moment, for literally anything.

And God. When it is just Esther and me in our bedroom, laying down for a nap or bedtime, God is there. He is in the calm and quiet as well as the upheaval and storm. He inhabits the deep recesses of my mind and brings true peace.

> *Isaiah 41:10: "Fear not, for I am with you; be not dismayed, for I am your God; I will strengthen you, I will help you, I will uphold you with my righteous right hand."*

More Experienced Parent

The more I mull over writing a book on this subject, the less qualified I feel to do so. Before Esther, my closest encounter with cancer was through my grandma—who I loved but never lived close to. I didn't know chemo. Or hospitals. Or the fear.

What is my level of hardship compared to so many others? What is my level of wisdom? (Hello, mother of one toddler here.) Who am I to say that my small revelations and advice are superior or new information to others? I speak to other moms in the trenches and hear the hope and pain and reality that tinges every aspect of life. I'm not going to be setting their worlds on fire with the words in this book: they already know.

But I had to write. I had to pour the words out of my heart and into this book so that maybe one or two moms would take courage and know they're not alone. That they would nod and smile and cry at my words that are all too familiar. We're all together in this lifeboat, rowing together and sharing snacks.

Little Baby Parent

Epilogue

This book ends, but cancer doesn't. Like the endless cares of motherhood, the threat of recurrence looms large.

I really, really don't want to write any sort of sequel to this book.

But life moves forward. Being in the cancer world is akin to riding a slow-moving conveyer belt, watching people finish the ride with quiet tears of deep-seeded joy, and seeing people get pushed onto it for the first time. It was a circle of life moment when I stepped outside myself and saw the progression. Our friend, Tommy, finished treatment. Then Ben. Then Henry. Port removal surgeries are scheduled every week, kids and parents rejoicing that this chapter in cancer is closed—hopefully never to be reprised.

But port placement surgeries are also scheduled every week. Tommy had his port put back in after less than a year, because the cancer was back. Folks new to the game are even more common. Wide-eyed parents and kids nodding to medical professionals, trying to catch their breath and catch up with this machine that drags them along until they can stumble unsteadily to their feet. Diagnosis, treatment plan, completion, repeat. Many live this cycle many times themselves, having their feet knocked out from under them, being shoved unceremoniously to the beginning of the conveyer belt when they thought they were already done, or nearing the end.

We all hope that it won't be us, making macabre jokes about being a frequent flier. We also hope it won't be our friends. Or that one kid we see once in a while but don't know their name. But it has to be someone. Why? Why does it have to be someone? Why not nobody? How about pediatric cancer just end? *Instead of causing ends.* Kids being slapped off the conveyer belt mid-journey. The gap they leave in their wake is easily seen in empty beds and the eyes of haunted parents. The treatment process isn't short or easy, but it's better than the alternative.

When I first found out I was pregnant with Esther, fear consumed me. *What if I miscarried? I'd feel better in a few months. When she was bigger. She's much more likely to make it to birth. But I guess that's not a forgone conclusion. OK, OK; let's just say I'll feel better when she's born. An 8 lb. 12 oz. baby is pretty bulletproof.* But, no, I realized. The fear wouldn't stop then. In fact, there would always be reasons to fear.

So in that moment, with a mustard-seed-sized Esther inside me, I made myself a promise that I would try not to be scared. I know bad things of every variety can happen, but being afraid in advance doesn't change reality. I would be thankful for every moment and try not to fear what I could not control. It's been a good goal to aspire to—one that I remind myself of almost daily.

You'll take your kid back to the cancer doctor for regular checkups for the rest of their childhood, and every blood test or scan result will have your heart racing. Your child will grow up and have their own family doctor. They will always have to check the "pediatric cancer" check box on their medical history form and continue to be regularly monitored.

You will be afraid sometimes. But live your life in hope, because it's not worth your time to ruin it in fear.

Faithful Reader,

Well done. You've made it to the end. Or you've skipped to the last few pages to see how it turns out. Wouldn't it be nice if that were the case in real life?

I've prayed over these words with every step, that they would be glorifying to God and helpful to you. Or at least one person in the world. Maybe that's you.

If you are interested in following along with Esther's cancer journey or joining with the prayer warrior task force, feel free to follow 'Praying for Baby Esther" on Facebook.

www.facebook.com/groups/prayingforbabyesther/

Or you're welcome to join if you're just desperately in need of up-to-date photos of my child, because let's face it, Esther is extremely adorable.

Thanks for reading. May God reveal Himself to you more intimately on whatever journey you're on.

Humbled Author

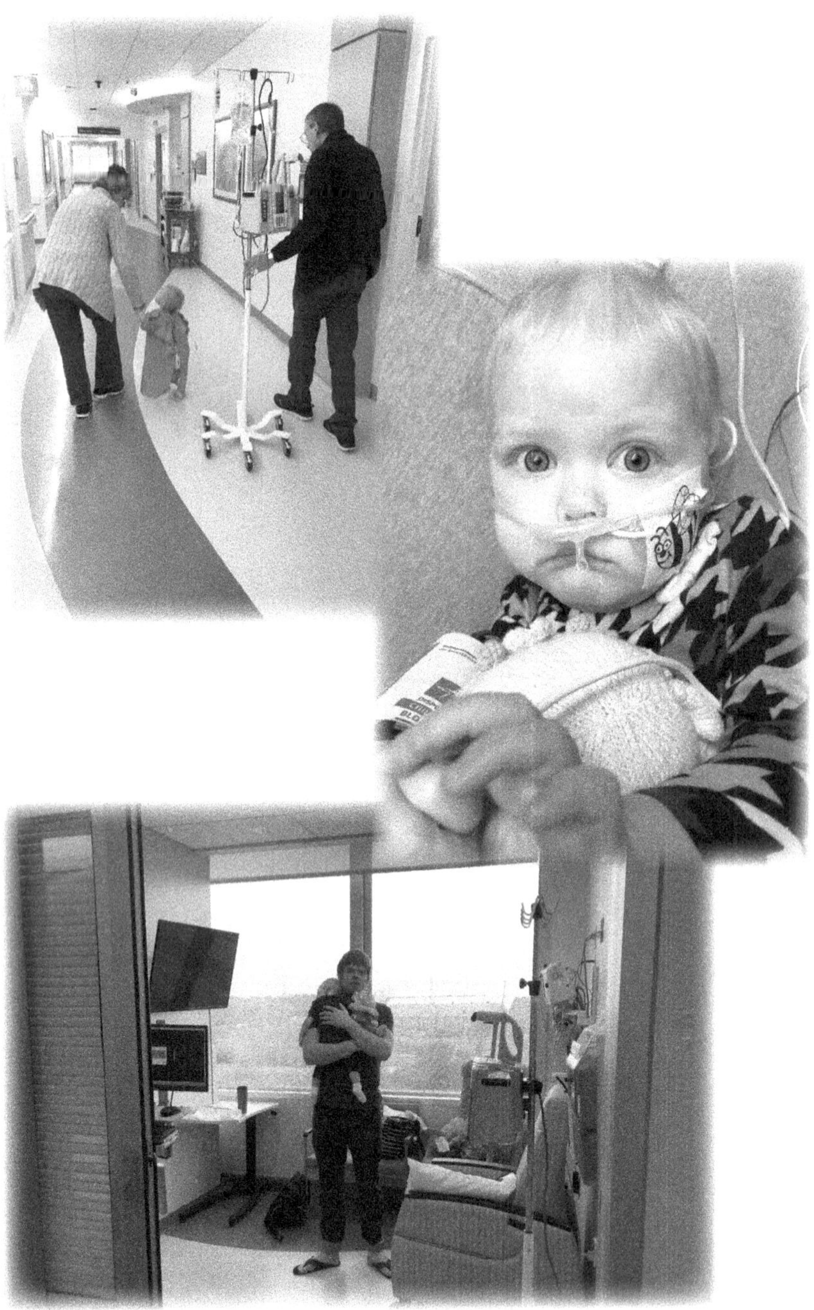

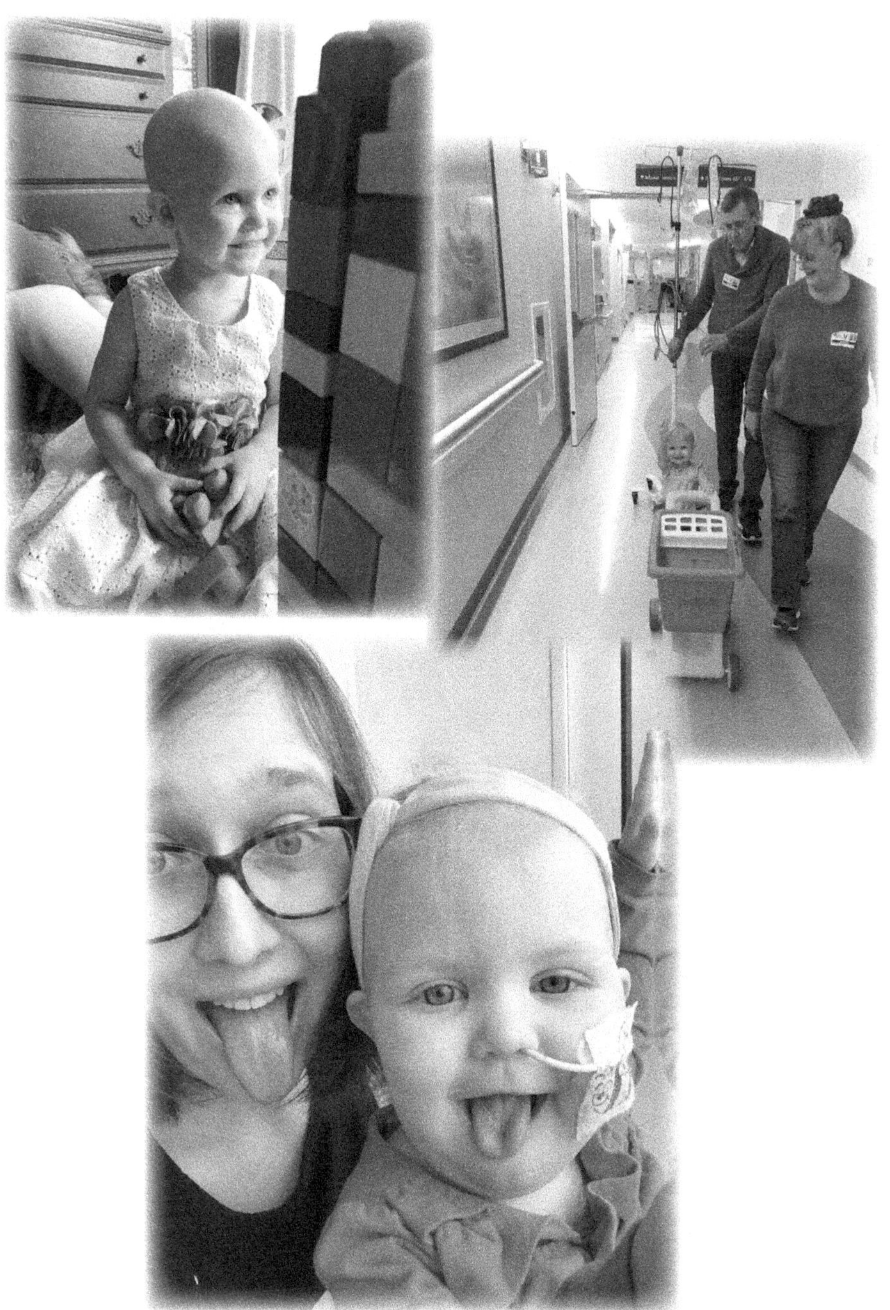

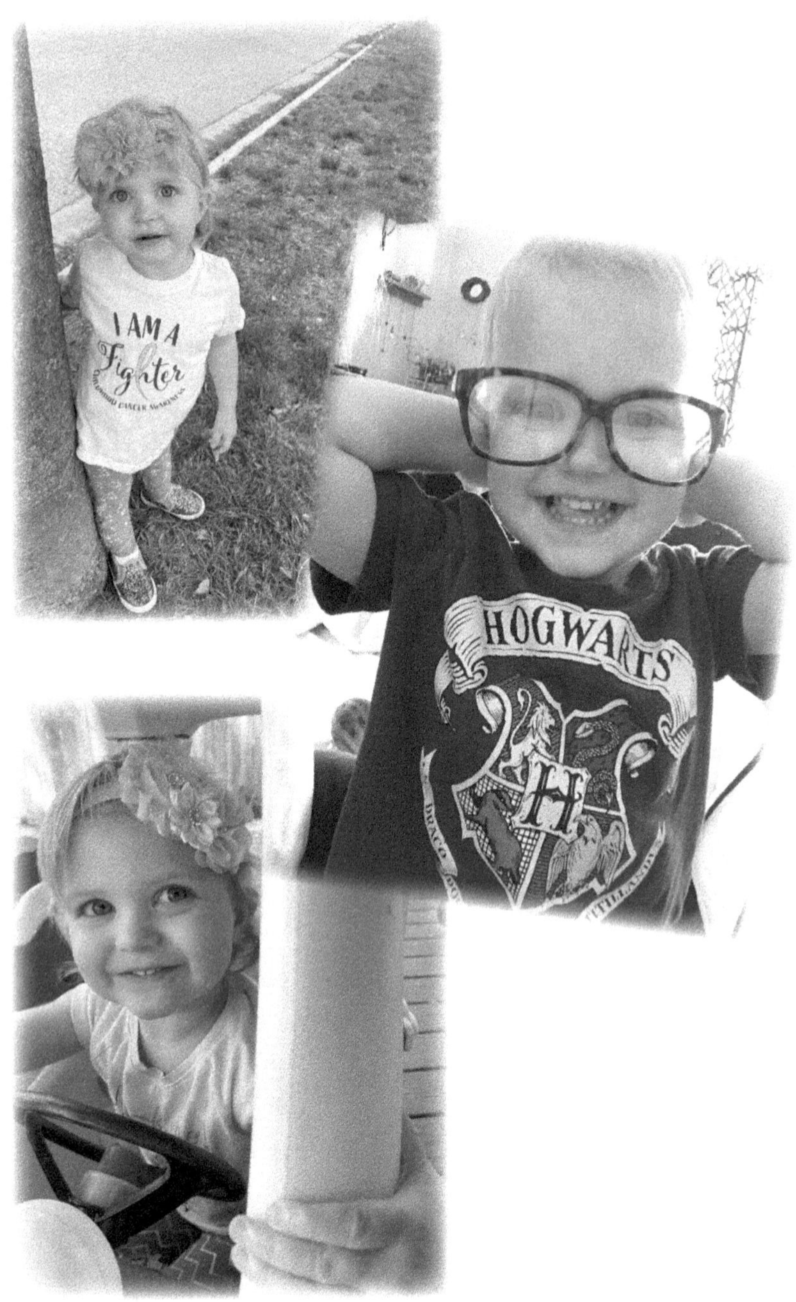
I AM A
Fighter
HOGWARTS

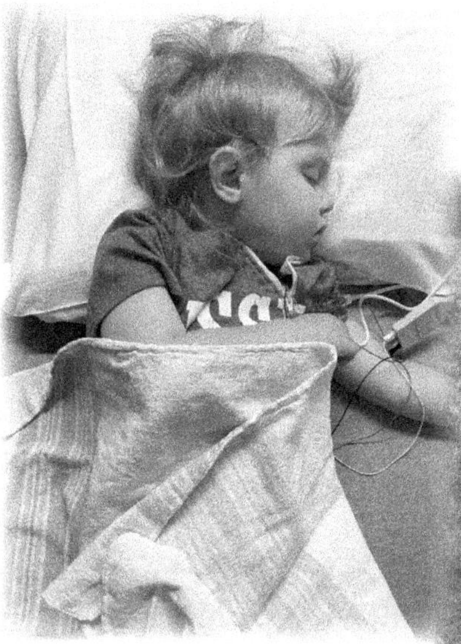

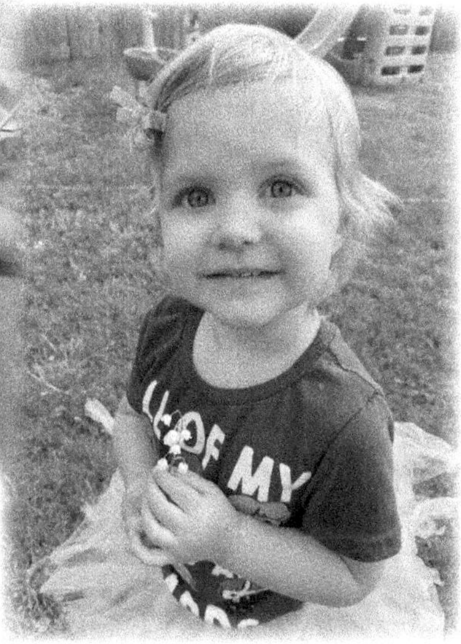

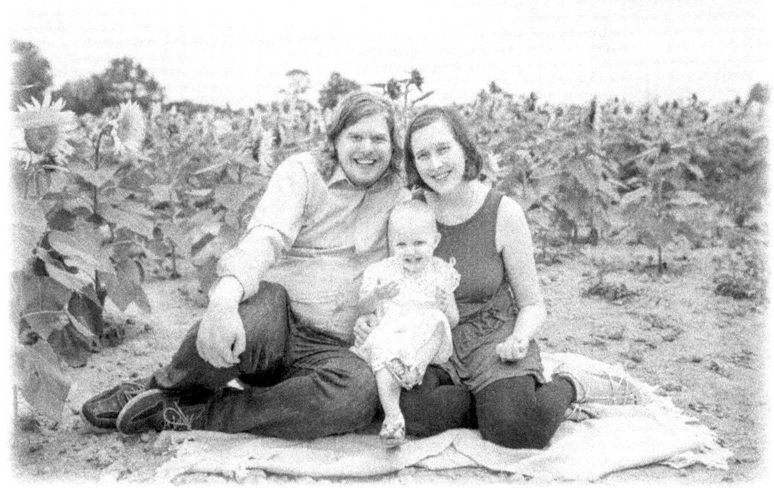

Photo by Karen Schanely Photography

Resources

MOMCOLOGY

103 Wellwood Avenue
Saint Johns, FL 32259
Email: info@momcology.org
momcology.org
facebook.com/ momcologyorg

CHILDREN'S ONCOLOGY GROUP

800 Royal Oaks Drive, Suite 210
Monrovia, CA 91016
Email: HelpDesk@childrensoncologygroup.org
childrensoncologygroup.org

NATIONAL CANCER INSTITUTE

Email: NCIinfo@nih.gov
cancer.gov

LA LECHE LEAGUE

110 Horizon Drive, Suite 210
Raleigh, NC 27615, USA
Email: info@llli.org
llli.org
La Leche League's: *The Womanly Art of Breastfeeding* by Diane Wiessinger, Diana West & and Teresa Pitman

www.ingramcontent.com/pod-product-compliance
Lightning Source LLC
Chambersburg PA
CBHW072125090426
42739CB00012B/3067

* 9 7 8 1 6 1 3 1 4 5 3 8 8 *